THE SIMPLE

KETOGENIC

DIET

THE ESSENTIAL FAT BURNING

FORMULA FOR ANY BODY

Mike Manes

Table of Contents

Chapter 1: Keto Basics

In the introduction we briefly discussed the meaning and theory behind ketogenic dieting. Here we will delve further into the science behind the method and how it can boost your metabolism and detox your body in 10 days.

Benefits of Increased Metabolism

One of the best ways to learn the meaning of a scientific term is to break it down to its roots. When we break down ketogenic we see it is comprised of two words: keto and genic. Ketones are fat-based molecules that the body breaks down when it is using fat as its energy source. When used as a suffix, "genic" means "causing, forming, or producing". So, we put these terms together and we have "ketogenic", or simply put, "causing fat burn". Ergo, the theory behind ketogenic dieting is: when a person reduces the amount of sugar and carbohydrates they consume, the body will begin to breakdown fat it already has in stores all over the body. When your body is cashing in on these stores, it is in a ketogenic state, or "ketosis". When your body consumes food, it naturally seeks carbohydrates for the purpose of breaking them down and using them as fuel. Adversely, a ketogenic cleanse trains your body to use fats for energy instead. This is achieved by lowering the amount of ingested carbohydrates and increasing the amount of ingested fats, which in turn boosts your metabolism.

Only recently has a low carb- high fat diet plan emerged into the public eye. It is a sharp contrast to the traditional dieting style that emphasizes calorie counting. For many years it was over looked that crash diets neglect the most important aspect of dieting: food is fuel. A diet is not meant be treated as a once a year go to method in order to shed holiday weight in January. Rather, a diet is a lifestyle; it is a consistent pattern of how an individual fuels their body. A ten day ketogenic cleanse is the perfect way to begin forming healthy eating habits that overtime become second nature. If you are tired of losing weight just to gain it all back, never fear. We firmly believe that you can accomplish anything you put your mind to, including living a healthy life! You, like hundreds of others, can successfully accomplish a ketogenic cleanse and change the way you see health, fitness, and life along the way. So let's hit the books and get that metabolism working!

Benefits of Cleansing

In addition to increased metabolism and fat loss, ketogenic cleansing allows your body naturally rid itself of harmful toxins and wasteful substances. In today's modern world, food is overrun and polluted by genetically modified hormones, artificial flavors and coloring, and copious amounts of unnecessary sugars. Ketogenic cleansing eliminates breads, grains, and many other foods that are most affected by today's modern industrialization. Due to the high amount of naturally occurring foods used in a ketogenic cleanse, the body is able to obtain many vitamins and minerals that are not prevalent in a high carb diet. When the body is consuming sufficient amounts of necessary vitamins and minerals, it is able to heal itself and maintain a healthy immune system. Cleansing your body is one of the best ways to achieve, and maintain, pristine health.

Chapter 2: Meal Plan Madness

One of the best ways to stay motivated, when dieting, is to find a meal plan that is easy to follow and easy on the budget. Ketogenic meals are designed to be filling while keeping within the perimeters of low-carb, high-fat guidelines. Ideally you want to aim for 70% fats, 25% protein, and 5% carbohydrates in your diet. As long as the materials you use to build your meals are low in carbs and high in fats, feel free to experiment and find what is right for you. Each and every one of us is different and that's okay. After all, this meal plan is for YOU!

Below is a ten day meal plan, designed with a busy schedule in mind, which will not break the bank! All of these meals can be prepared in 30 minutes or less, and many of them are much quicker than that! There is also a list of ingredients for each meal located in the recipe chapter so you can go to the grocery store knowing exactly what you need!

	Breakfast	Lunch	Dinner

Day 1	California Chicken Omelet • Fat: 32 grams • 10 minutes to prepare • Protein: 25 grams • 10 minutes of cooking • Net carbs: 4 grams	Cobb Salad • Fat: 48 grams • 10 minutes to prepare • Protein: 43 grams • 0 minutes of cooking • Net carbs: 3 grams	Chicken Peanut Pad Thai • Fat: 12 grams • 15 minutes to prepare • Protein: 30 grams • 15 minutes of cooking • Net carbs: 2 grams
Day 2	Easy Blender Pancakes • Fat: 29 grams • 5 minutes to prepare • Protein: 41 grams • 10 minutes of cooking • Net carbs: 4 grams	Sardine Stuffed Avocados • Fat: 29 grams • 10 minutes to prepare • Protein: 27 grams • 0 minutes of cooking • Net Carbs: 5 grams	Chipotle Fish Tacos • Fat: 20 grams • 5 minutes to prepare • Protein: 24 grams • 15 minutes of cooking • Net carbs: 5 grams
Day 3	Steak and Eggs • Fat: 36 grams • 10 minutes to prepare • Protein: 47 grams • 5 minutes of cooking • Net carbs: 3 grams	Low-Carb Smoothie Bowl • Fat 35 grams • 5 minutes to prepare • Protein: 20 grams • 0 minutes of cooking • Net carbs: 5 grams	Avocado Lime Salmon • Fat: 27 grams • 20 minutes to prepare • Protein: 37 grams • 10 minutes of cooking • Net carbs: 5 grams
	During the course of your plan, especially around days 3 and 4, you may begin to feel like you don't have it in you. You may have thoughts telling you that you cannot last for ten days on this type pf cleanse. Do not allow feelings of discouragement bother you because, guess what? We		

THE SIMPLE KETOGENIC DIET

KEEP IT UP!!!	all feel that way sometimes! A ketogenic diet causes your body to process energy like it never has before. Keep pressing on! Your body will thank you and so will you!		
Day 4	**Low-Carb Smoothie Bowl** • Fat: 35 grams • 5 minutes to prepare • Protein: 35 grams • 0 minutes of cooking • Net carbs: 4 grams	**Pesto Chicken Salad** • Fat: 27 grams • 5 minutes to prepare • Protein: 27 grams • 10 minutes of cooking • Net carbs: 3 grams	**Siracha Lime Flank Steak** • Fat: 32 grams • 5 minutes to prepare • Protein: 48 grams • 10 minutes of cooking • Net Carbs: 5 grams
Day 5	**Feta and Pesto Omelet** • Fat: 46 grams • 5 minutes of preparation • Protein: 30 grams • 5 minutes of cooking • Net carbs: 2.5 grams	**Roasted Brussel Sprouts** • Fat: 21 grams • 5 minutes to prepare • Protein: 21 grams • 30 minutes of cooking • Net carbs: 4 grams	**Low carb Sesame Chicken** • Fat: 36 grams • 15 minutes to prepare • Protein: 41 grams • 15 minutes of cooking • Net carbs: 4 grams
Day 6	**Raspberry Cream Crepes** • Fat: 40 grams • 5 minutes of preparation • Net carbs: 8 grams • 15 minutes of cooking • Protein 15 grams	**Shakshuka** • Fat: 34 grams • Protein 35 grams • Net carbs: 4 grams • 10 minutes of preparation • 10 minutes of cooking	**Sausage in a Pan** • Fat: 38 grams • 10 minutes of preparation • Protein: 30 grams • 25 minutes of cooking • Net Carbs: 4 grams

Day 7	Green Monster Smoothie	Tuna Tartare	Pesto Chicken Salad
	• Fat: 25 grams • 5 minutes of preparation • Protein: 30 grams • 0 minutes of cooking • Net Carbs: 3 grams	• Fat: 24 grams • 15 minutes of preparation • Protein: 56 grams • 0 minutes of cooking • Net Carbs: 4 grams	• Fat: 27 grams • 5 minutes of preparation • Protein: 27 grams • 10 minutes of cooking • Net carbs: 3 grams
ALMOST THERE!!	By now, you can be certain you are seeing physical results such as reduced body fat and more energy! You are doing a fantastic job and you only have three days left! Keep up the good work, you owe it to yourself.		
Day 8	Shakshuka	Grilled Halloumi Salad	Keto Quarter Pounder
	• Fat: 34 grams • 10 minutes of preparation • Protein 35 grams • 10 minutes of cooking • Net carbs: 4 grams	• Fat: 47 grams • 15 minutes of preparation • Protein: 21 grams • 0 minutes of cooking • Net carbs: 2 grams	• Fat: 34 grams • 10 minutes of preparation • Protein: 25 grams • 8 minutes of cooking • Net carbs: 4 •
Day 9	Easy Blender Pancakes	Broccoli Bacon Salad	Sardine Stuffed Avocados
	• Fat: 29 grams • 5 minutes of preparation • Protein: 41 grams • 10 minutes of cooking • Net carbs: 4 grams	• Fat: 31 grams • 15 minutes of preparation • Protein: 10 grams • 6 minutes of cooking	• Fat: 29 grams • 10 minutes to prepare • Protein: 27 grams • 0 minutes to cook

		• Net carbs: 5 grams	• Net Carbs: 5 grams
Day 10	**California Chicken Omelet** • Fat 32 grams • 10 minutes to prepare • Protein 25 grams • 10 minutes of cooking • Net carb: 3 grams	**Shrimp Scampi** • Fat: 21 grams • 5 minutes to prepare • Protein: 21 grams • 30 minutes of cooking • Net carbs: 4 grams	**Tuna Tartare** • Fat: 36 grams • 15 minutes to prepare • Protein: 41 grams • 15 minutes of cooking • Net carbs: 4 grams
YOU DID IT!!	Congratulations! You have successfully completed a 10 day ketogenic cleanse. By now your body has adjusted to its new source of energy, expelled dozens of harmful toxins, and replenished itself with many vitamins and minerals it may have been lacking. Way to go on a job well done!		

Chapter 3: Breakfast Is For Champions

Breakfast is by far the most important meal of the day for one reason: it set the tone for the rest of your day. In order to hit the ground running, it is vital that one starts each day with foods that fuel an energetic and productive day. This chapter contains ten ketogenic breakfast ides that will have you burning fat and conquering your day like you never imagined.

1. California Chicken Omelet

- This recipe requires 10 minutes of preparation, 10 minutes of cooking time and serves 1
- Net carbs: 4 grams

- Protein: 25 grams

- Fat : 32 grams

What you will need:

- Mayo (1 tablespoon)

- Mustard (1 teaspoon)

- Campari tomato

- Eggs (2 large beaten)

- Avocado (one fourth, sliced)

- Bacon (2 slices cooked and chopped)

- Deli chicken (1 ounce)

What to do:

1. Place a skillet on the stove over a burner set to a medium heat and let it warm before adding in the eggs and seasoning as needed.

2. Once eggs are cooked about halfway through, add bacon, chicken, avocado, tomato, mayo, and mustard on one side of the eggs.

3. Fold the omelet onto its self, cover and cook for 5 additional minutes.

4. Once eggs are fully cooked and all ingredients are warm, through the center, your omelet is ready.

5. Bon apatite!

2. Steak and Eggs with Avocado

- This recipe requires 10 minutes of preparation, 5 minutes of cooking time and serves 1

- Net Carbs: 3 grams

- Protein: 44 grams

- Fat: 36 grams

What you will need:

- Salt and pepper
- Avocado (one fourth, sliced)
- Sirloin steak (4 ounce)
- Eggs (3 large)
- Butter (1 tablespoon)

What to do:

1. Melt the tablespoon of butter in a pan and fry all 3 eggs to desired doneness. Season the eggs with salt and pepper.

2. In a different pan, cook the sirloin steak to your preferred taste and slice it into thin strips. Season the steak with salt and pepper.

3. Sever your prepared steak and eggs with slices of avocado.

4. Enjoy!

3. Pancakes an a Blender

- This recipe requires 5 minutes of preparation, 10 minutes of cooking time and serves 1
- Net Carbs: 4 grams
- Protein: 41 grams
- Fat: 29 grams

What you will need:

- Whey protein powder (1 scoop)
- Eggs (2 large)
- Cream cheese (2 ounces)
- Just a pinch of cinnamon and a pinch of salt

What to do:

1. Combine cream cheese, eggs, protein powder, cinnamon, and salt into a blender. Blend for 10 seconds and let stand.
2. While letting batter stand, warm a skillet over medium heat.
3. Pour about ¼ of the batter onto warmed skillet and let cook. When bubbles begin to emerge on the surface, flip the pancake.
4. Once flipped, cook for 15 seconds. Repeat until remainder of the batter is used up.
5. Top with butter and/ or sugar- free maple syrup and you are all set!
6. Chow time!

4. Low Carb Smoothe Bowl

- Net Carbs: 4 grams

- Protein: 35 grams

- Fat: 35 grams

- Takes 5 minutes to prepare and serves 1.

What you will need:

- Spinach (1 cup)

- Almond milk (half a cup)

- Coconut oil (1 tablespoon)

- Low carb protein powder (1 scoop)

- Ice cubes (2 cubes)

- Whipping cream (2 T)

- Optional toppings can include: raspberries, walnuts, shredded coconut, or chia seeds

What to do:

1. Place spinach in blender. Add almond milk, cream, coconut oil, and ice. Blend until thoroughly and evenly combined.

2. Pour into bowl.

3. Top with toppings or stir lightly into smoothie.

4. Treat yourself!

THE SIMPLE KETOGENIC DIET

5. Feta and Pesto Omelet

- This recipe requires 5 minutes of preparation, 5 minutes of cooking time and serves 1
- Net Carbs: 2.5 grams
- Protein: 30 grams
- Fat: 46 grams

What you will need:

- Butter (1 tablespoon)
- Eggs (3 large)
- Heavy cream (1 tablespoon)
- Feta cheese (1 ounce)
- Basil pesto (1 teaspoon)
- Tomatoes (optional)

What to do:

1. Heat pan and melt butter.
2. Beat eggs together with heavy whipping cream (will give eggs a fluffy consistency once cooked).
3. Pour eggs in pan and cook until almost done, add feta and pesto to on half of eggs.
4. Fold omelet and cook for an additional 4-5 minutes.
5. Top with feta and tomatoes, and eat up!

6. Crepes with Cream and Raspberries

- This recipe requires 5 minutes of preparation, 15 minutes of cooking time and serves 2

- Net Carbs: 8 grams

- Protein: 15 grams

- Fat: 40 grams

What you will need:

- Raspberries (3 ounces, fresh or frozen)
- Whole Milk Ricotta (half a cup and 2 tablespoons)
- Erythritol (2 tablespoons)
- Eggs (2 large)
- Cream Cheese (2 ounces)
- Pinch of salt
- Dash of Cinnamon
- Whipped cream and sugar- free maple syrup to go on top

What to do:

1. In a blender, blend cream cheese, eggs, erythritol, salt, and cinnamon for about 20 seconds, or until there are no lumps of cream cheese.

2. Place a pan on a burner turned to a medium heat before coating in cooking spray. Add 20 percent of your batter to the pan in a thin layer. Cook crepe until the underside becomes slightly darkened. Carefully flip the crepe and let the reverse side cook for about 15 seconds.

3. Repeat step 3 until all batter is used.

4. Without stacking the crepes, allow them to cool for a few minutes.

5. After the crepes have cool, place about 2 tablespoons of ricotta cheese in the center of each crepe.

6. Throw in a couple of raspberries and fold the side to the middle.

7. Top those off with some whipped cream and sugar- free maple syrup and…

8. Viola! You're a true chef! Indulge in your creation!

7. Green Monster Smoothie

- This recipe requires 10 minutes of preparation, 0 minutes of cooking time and serves 1
- Net Carbs: 4 grams
- Protein: 30 grams
- Fat: 25 grams

What you will need:

- Almond milk (one and a half cups)
- Spinach (one eighth of a cup)
- Cucumber (fourth of a cup)
- Celery (fourth of a cup)
- Avocado (fourth of a cup)
- Coconut oil (1 tablespoon)
- Stevia (liquid, 10 drops)
- Whey Protein Powder (1 scoop)

What to do:

1. In a blender, blend almond milk and spinach for a few pulses.

2. Add remaining ingredients and blend until thoroughly combined.

• Add optional matcha powder, if desired, and enjoy!

Chapter 4: Lunch Crunch

Eating a healthy lunch when you are limited on time due to, work, school, or taking care of your kids can be a tumultuous task. Thankfully, we have compiled a list of eight quick and easy recipes to accompany the ten day meal plan laid out in chapter 2! Many find it advantageous, especially if you work throughout the week, to prepare you meals ahead of time. Thankfully, these lunch recipes are also easy to pack and take on the go!

1. Off The Cobb Salad

- Net carbs: 3 grams
- Protein: 43 grams
- Fat: 48 grams
- Takes 10 minutes to prepare and serves 1.

What you will need:

- Spinach (1 cup)
- Egg (1, hard-boiled)
- Bacon (2 strips)
- Chicken breast (2 ounces)
- Campari tomato (one half of tomato)
- Avocado (one fourth, sliced)
- White vinegar (half of a teaspoon)
- Olive oil (1 tablespoon)

What to do:

1. Cook chicken and bacon completely and cut or slice into small pieces.

2. Chop remaining ingredients into bite size pieces.

3. Place all ingredients, including chicken and bacon, in a bowl, toss ingredients in oil and vinegar.

4. Enjoy!

2. Avocado and Sardines

- Net Carbs: 5 grams
- Protein: 27 grams
- Fat: 52 grams
- Takes 10 minutes to prepare and serves 1.

What you will need:

- Fresh lemon juice (1 tablespoon)
- Spring onion or chives (1 or small bunch)
- Mayonnaise (1 tablespoon)
- Sardines (1 tin, drained)
- Avocado (1 whole, seed removed)
- Turmeric powder (fourth of a teaspoon) or freshly ground turmeric root (1 teaspoon)
- Salt (fourth of a teaspoon)

What to do:

1. Begin by cutting the avocado in half and removing its seed.

2. Scoop out about half the avocado and set aside (shown below).

3. In small bowl, mash drained sardines with fork.

4. Add onion (or chives), turmeric powder, and mayonnaise. Mix well.

5. Add removed avocado to sardine mixture.

6. Add lemon juice and salt.

7. Scoop the mixture into avocado halves.

8. Dig in!

3. Chicken Salad A La Pesto

- This recipe requires 5minutes of preparation, 10 minutes of cooking time and serves 4

- Net Carbs: 3 grams

- Protein: 27 grams

- Fat: 27 grams

What you will need:

- Garlic pesto (2 tablespoons)

- Mayonnaise (fourth of a cup)

- Grape tomatoes (10, halved)

- Avocado (1, cubed)

- Bacon (6 slices, cooked crisp and crumbled)

- Chicken (1 pound, cooked and cubed)

- Romaine lettuce (optional)

What to do:

1. Combine all ingredients in a large mixing bowl.

2. Toss gently to spread mayonnaise and pesto evenly throughout.

3. If desired, wrap in romaine lettuce for a low-carb BLT chicken wrap.

4. Bon apatite!

4. Bacon and Roasted Brussel Sprouts

- This recipe requires 5 minutes of preparation, 30 minutes of cooking time and serves 4
- Net Carbs: 4 grams
- Protein: 15 grams
- Fat: 21 grams

What you will need:

- Bacon (8 strips)
- Olive oil (2 tablespoons)
- Brussel sprouts (1 pound, halved)
- Salt and pepper

What to do:

1. Preheat oven to 375 degrees Fahrenheit.
2. Gently mix Brussel sprouts with olive oil, salt, and pepper.
3. Spread Brussel sprouts evenly onto a greased baking sheet.
4. Bake in oven for 30 minutes. Shake the pan about halfway through to mix the Brussel sprout halves up a bit.

5. While Brussel sprouts are in the oven, fry bacon slices on stovetop.

6. When bacon is fully cooked, let cool and chop it into bite size pieces.

7. Combine bacon and Brussel sprouts in a bowl and you're finished!

8. Feast!!

5. Grilled Halloumi Salad

- Net Carbs: 7 grams
- Protein: 21 grams
- Fat: 47 grams
- Takes 15 minutes to prepare and serves 1.

What you will need:

- Chopped walnuts (half of an ounce)
- Baby arugula (1 handful)
- Grape tomatoes (5)
- Cucumber (1)
- Halloumi cheese (3 ounces)
- Olive oil (1 teaspoon)
- Balsamic vinegar (half of a teaspoon)
- A pinch of salt

What to do:

1. Slice halloumi cheese into slices 1/3 of an in thick.

2. Grill cheese for 3 to 5 minutes, until you see grill lines, on each side.

3. Wash and cut veggies into bite size pieces, place in salad bowl.

4. Add rinsed baby arugula and walnuts to veggies.

5. Toss in olive oil, balsamic vinegar, and salt.

6. Place grilled halloumi on top of veggies and your lunch is ready!

7. Eat those greens and get back to work!

6. Bacon Broccoli Salad

- This recipe requires 15 minutes of preparation, 6 minutes of cooking time and serves 5.
- Net Carbs: 5 grams
- Protein: 10 grams
- Fat: 31 grams

What you will need:

- Sesame oil (half of a teaspoon)
- Erythritol (1 and a half tablespoons) or stevia to taste
- White vinegar (1 tablespoon)
- Mayonnaise (half of a cup)
- Green onion (three fourths of an ounce)
- Bacon (fourth of a pound)

- Broccoli (1 pound, heads and stalks cut and trimmed)

What to do:

1. Cook bacon and crumble into bits.
2. Cut broccoli into bite sized pieces.
3. Slice scallions.
4. Mix mayonnaise, vinegar, erythritol (or stevia), and sesame oil, to make the dressing.
5. Place broccoli and bacon bits in a bowl and toss with dressing.
6. Viola!

7. Tuna Avocado Tartare

- Net Carbs: 4 grams
- Protein: 56 grams
- Fat: 24 grams
- Takes 15 minutes to prepare and serves 2.

What you will need:

- Sesame seed oil (2 tablespoons)
- Sesame seeds (1 teaspoon)
- Cucumbers (2)
- Lime (half of a whole lime)
- Mayonnaise (1 tablespoon)
- Sriracha (1 tablespoon)
- Olive oil (2 tablespoons)
- Jalapeno (one half of whole jalapeno)
- Scallion (3 stalks)

- Avocado (1)
- Tuna steak (1 pound)
- Soy sauce (1 tablespoon)

What to do:

1. Dice tuna and avocado into ¼ inch cubes, place in bowl.

2. Finely chop scallion and jalapeno, add to bowl.

3. Pour olive oil, sesame oil, siracha, soy sauce, mayonnaise, and lime into bowl.

4. Using hands, toss all ingredients to combine evenly. Using a utensil may breakdown avocado, which you want to remain chunky, so it is best to use your hands.

5. Top with sesame seeds and serve with a side of sliced cucumber.

6. There's certainly something fishy about this recipe, but it tastes great! Enjoy!

8. Warm Spinach and Shrimp

- This recipe requires 15 minutes of preparation, 6 minutes of cooking time and serves 5.

- Fat: 24 grams

- Protein: 36 grams

- Net Carbs: 3 grams

- Takes 10 minutes to prepare, 5 minutes to cook, and serves 2.

What you will need:

- Spinach (2 handfuls)

- Parmesan (half a tablespoon)

- Heavy cream (1 tablespoon)

- Olive oil (1 tablespoon)

- Butter (2 tablespoons)

- Garlic (3 cloves)

- Onion (one fourth of whole onion)

- Large raw shrimp (about 20)

- Lemon (optional)

What to do:

1. Place peeled shrimp in cold water.

2. Chop onions and garlic into fine pieces.

3. Heat oil, in pan, over medium heat. Cook shrimp in oil until lightly pink (we do not want them fully cooked here). Remove shrimp from oil and set aside.

4. Place chopped onions and garlic into pan, cook until onions are translucent. Add a dash of salt.

5. Add butter, cream, and parmesan cheese. Stir until you have a smooth sauce.

6. Let sauce cook for about 2 minutes so it will thicken slightly.

7. Place shrimp back into pan and cook until done. This should take no longer than 2 or 3 minutes. Be careful not to overcook the shrimp, it will become dry and tough!

8. Remove shrimp and sauce from pan and replace with spinach. Cook spinach VERY briefly

9. Place warmed spinach onto a plate.

10. Pour shrimp and sauce over bed of spinach, squeeze some lemon on top, if you like, and you're ready to chow down!

Chapter 5: Thinner by Dinner

It's the end of the day and you are winding down from a hard day's work. Your body does not require a lot of energy while you sleep; therefore, dinner will typically consist of less fat and more protein.

1. Chicken Pad Thai

- Net Carbs: 7 grams
- Protein: 30 grams
- Fat: 12 grams
- Takes 15 minutes to prepare, 15 minutes to cook, and serves 4.

What you will need:

- Peanuts (1 ounce)
- Lime (1 whole)
- Soy sauce (2 tablespoons)
- Egg (1 large)
- Zucchini (2 large)
- Chicken thighs (16 ounces, boneless and skinless)
- Garlic (2 cloves, minced)
- White onion (1,chopped)
- Olive oil (1 tablespoon)
- Chili flakes (optional)

What to do:

1. Over medium heat, cook olive oil and onion until translucent. Add the garlic and cook about three minutes (until fragrant).

2. Cook chicken in pan for 5 to 7 minutes on each side (until fully cooked). Remove chicken from heat and shred it using a couple of forks.

3. Cut ends off zucchini and cut into thin noodles. Set zucchini noodles aside.

4. Next, scramble the egg in the pan.

5. Once the egg is fully cooked, and the zucchini noodles and cook for about 2 minutes.

6. Add the previously shredded chicken to the pan.

7. Give it some zing with soy sauce, lime juice, peanuts, and chili flakes.

8. Time to eat!

2. Chipotle Style Fish Tacos

- Fat: 20 grams
- Protein: 24 grams
- Net Carbs: 7 grams
- Takes 5 minutes to prepare, 15 minutes to cook, and serves 4.

What you will need:

- Low carb tortillas (4)

- Haddock fillets (1 pound)

- Mayonnaise (2 tablespoons)

- Butter (2 tablespoons)

- Chipotle peppers in adobo sauce (4 ounces)

- Garlic (2 cloves, pressed)

- Jalapeño (1 fresh, chopped)

- Olive oil (2 tablespoons)

- Yellow onion (half of an onion, diced)

What to do:

1. Fry diced onion (until translucent) in olive oil in a high sided pan, over medium- high heat.

2. Reduce heat to medium, add jalapeno and garlic. Cook while stir for another two minutes.

3. Chop the chipotle peppers and add them, along with the adobo sauce, to the pan.

4. Add the butter, mayo, and fish fillets to the pan.

5. Cook the fish fully while breaking up the fillets and stirring the fish into other ingredients.

6. Warm tortillas for 2 minutes on each side.

7. Fill tortillas with fishy goodness and eat up!

3. Salmon with Avocado Lime Sauce

- Net Carbs: 5 grams

- Protein: 37 grams

- Fat: 27 grams

- Takes 20 minutes to prepare, 10 minutes to cook, and serves 2.

What you will need:

- Salmon (two 6 ounce fillets)
- Avocado (1 large)
- Lime (one half of a whole lime)
- Red onion (2 tablespoons, diced)
- Cauliflower (100 grams)

What to do:

1. Chop cauliflower in a blender or food processor then cook it in a lightly oiled pan, while covered, for 8 minutes. This will make the cauliflower rice-like.

2. Next, blend the avocado with squeezed lime juice in the blender or processor until smooth and creamy.

3. Heat some oil in a skillet and cook salmon (skin side down first) for 4 to 5 minute. Flip the fillets and cook for an additional 4 to 5 minutes.

4. Place salmon fillet on a bed of your cauliflower rice and top with some diced red onion.

4. Siracha Lime Steak

- Net Carbs: 5 grams

- Protein: 48 grams

- Fat: 32 grams

- Takes 5 minutes to prepare, 10 minutes to cook, and serves 2.

What you will need:

- Vinegar (1 teaspoon)
- Olive oil (2 tablespoons)
- Lime (1 whole)
- Sriracha (2 tablespoons)
- Flank steak (16 ounce)
- Salt and pepper

What to do:

1. Season steak, liberally, with salt and pepper. Place on baking sheet, lined with foil, and broil in oven for 5 minutes on each side (add another minute or two for a well done steak). Remove from oven, cover, and set aside.
2. Place sriracha in small bowl and squeeze lime into it. Whisk in salt, pepper, and vinegar.
3. Slowly pour in olive oil.
4. Slice steak into thin slices, lather on your sauce, and enjoy!
5. Feel free to pair this recipe with a side of greens such as asparagus or broccoli.

5. Low Carb Sesame Chicken

- Net Carbs: 4 grams

- Protein: 45 grams

- Fat: 36 grams

- Takes 15minutes to prepare, 15 minutes to cook, and serves 2.

What you will need:

- Broccoli (three fourths of a cup, cut bite size)
- Xanthan gum (fourth of a teaspoon)
- Sesame seeds (2 tablespoons)
- Garlic (1 clove)
- Ginger (1 cm cube)
- Vinegar (1 tablespoon)
- Brown sugar alternative (Sukrin Gold is a good one) (2 tablespoons)
- Soy sauce (2 tablespoons)
- Toasted sesame seed oil (2 tablespoons)
- Arrowroot powder or corn starch (1 tablespoon)
- Chicken thighs (1poundcut into bite sized pieces)
- Egg (1 large)
- Salt and pepper
- Chives (optional)

What to do:

1. First we will make the batter by combining the egg with a tablespoon of arrowroot powder (or cornstarch). Whisk well.
2. Place chicken pieces in batter. Be sure to coat all sides of chicken pieces with the batter.

3. Heat one tablespoon of sesame oil, in a large pan. Add chicken pieces to hot oil and fry. Be gentle when flipping the chicken, you want to keep the batter from falling off. It should take about 10 minutes for them to cook fully.

4. Next, make the sesame sauce. In a small bowl, combine soy sauce, brown sugar alternative, vinegar, ginger, garlic, sesame seeds, and the remaining tablespoon of toasted sesame seed oil. Whisk very well.

5. Once the chicken is fully cooked, add broccoli and the sesame sauce to pan and cook for an additional 5 minutes.

6. Spoon desired amount into a bowl, top it off with some chopped chives, and relish in some fine dining at home!

6. Pan 'O Sausage

- Net Carbs: 4 grams

- Protein: 30 grams

- Fat: 38 grams

- Takes 10 minutes to prepare, 25 minutes to cook, and serves 2.

What you will need:

- Basil (half a teaspoon)

- Oregano (half a teaspoon)

- White onion (1 tablespoon)

- Shredded mozzarella (fourth of a cup)

- Parmesan cheese (fourth of a cup)

- Vodka sauce (half a cup)

- Mushrooms (4 ounces)

- Sausage (3 links)

- Salt (fourth of a teaspoon)

- Red pepper (fourth of a teaspoon, ground)

What to do:

1. Preheat oven to 350 degrees Fahrenheit.

2. Heat an iron skillet over medium flame. When skillet is hot, cook sausage links until almost thoroughly cooked.

3. While sausage is cooking, slice mushrooms and onion.

4. When sausage is almost fully cooked, remove links from heat and place mushrooms and onions in skillet to brown.

5. Cut sausage into pieces about ½ inch thick and place pieces in pan.

6. Season skillet contents with oregano, basil, salt, and red pepper.

7. Add vodka sauce and parmesan cheese. Stir everything together.

8. Place skillet in oven for 15 minutes. Sprinkle mozzarella on top a couple minutes before removing dish from oven.

9. Once 15 minutes is up, remove skillet from the oven and let cool for a few minutes.

10. Dinner time!

7. Quarter Pounder Keto Burger

- Net Carbs: 4 grams

- Protein: 25 grams

- Fat: 34 grams

- Takes 10 minutes to prepare, 8 minutes to cook, and serves 2.

What you will need:

- Basil (half a teaspoon)

- Cayenne (fourth a teaspoon)

- Crushed red pepper (half a teaspoon)

- Salt (half a teaspoon)

- Lettuce (2 large leaves)

- Butter (2 tablespoons)

- Egg (1 large)

- Sriracha (1 tablespoon)

- Onion (fourth of whole onion)

- Plum tomato (half of whole tomato)

- Mayo (1 tablespoon)

- Pickled jalapenos (1 tablespoon, sliced)

- Bacon (1 strip)

- Ground beef (half a pound)

- Bacon (1 strip)

What to do:

1. Knead mean for about three minute.

2. Chop bacon, jalapeno, tomato, and onion into fine pieces. (shown below)

3. Knead in mayo, sriracha, egg, and chopped ingredients, and spices into meat.

4. Separate meat into four even pieces and flatten them (not thinly, just press on the tops to create a flat surface). Place a tablespoon of butter on top of two of the meat pieces. Take the pieces that do not have butter of them and set them on top of the buttered ones (basically creating a butter and meat sandwich). Seal the sides together, concealing the butter within.

5. Throw the patties on the grill (or in a pan) for about 5 minutes on each side. Caramelize some onions if you want too!

6. Prepare large leaves of lettuce by spreading some mayo onto them. Once patties are finished, place them on one half of the lettuce, add your desired burger toppings, and fold the other half over of the lettuce leaf over the patty.

Burger time!

PART 2

Chapter 1: What Is the DASH Effect?

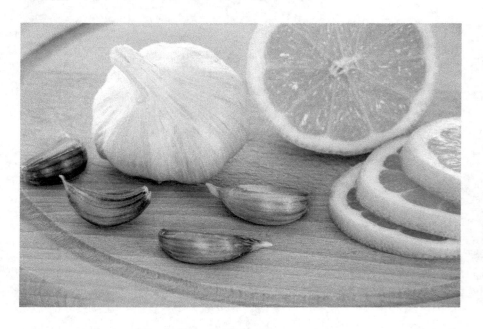

Are you suffering from hypertension? Do you need a great way to lower your sodium intake without losing the flavor in your meals? If you are searching for the most successful diet plan, then this is your book. The DASH effect diet was ranked the best diet for 7 years in a row by the United States News and World Report. If you've been looking for a weight loss program, then the DASH effect is exactly what you need.

The DASH effect diet is a diet designed to help reduce hypertension and lower blood pressure by providing a diet of clean, fresh foods with lots of color variety. By lowering your sodium intake, you can lower your blood pressure. It's also known to lower your blood sugar which makes it great for diabetics. So what is the DASH effect? Well,

DASH is an acronym for 'Dietary Approaches to Stop Hypertension.' With many Americans suffering from hypertension, having a healthy diet full of fresh, clean foods is something that everyone needs.

Since the DASH effect started, it has been making headlines. It is promoted by the National Heart, Lung and Blood Institute for hypertension and blood pressure. The USDA says that the DASH effect is the ideal plan for Americans, and the Kidney Foundation has endorsed it for people suffering from kidney disease. With endorsements like these, why is everyone not following the DASH effect diet plan? The true answer is that change is hard. But the DASH effect diet doesn't have to be.

So what exactly is the DASH effect and how can you incorporate it into your life? Well, that is really quite easy. Since most of you are already eating the key foods in the DASH effect, it should not be much of a drastic change. I think the biggest change is the lower sodium intake. You see, in a normal American diet, we consume around 3,500mg of sodium per day. In the DASH effect diet plan, we want to lower our sodium intake. So why should we do that? Lowering our sodium intake to either 2,300mg per day or 1,500mg per day can make changes that will transform our health.

By lowering our sodium we can remedy our hypertension, also known as 'blood pressure,' and even reduce our systolic blood pressure. But that isn't all, we can also reduce blood sugar levels, and it aids in preventing osteoporosis, cancer, stroke, and diabetes. The added reward is by reducing our sodium intake and eating a cleaner more natural diet we are also reducing our caloric intake and thus by reducing our weight. Even though weight loss is not the reason for this dietary plan, it is an added benefit. Everyone is interested in losing weight and with the DASH effect diet you can do just that without missing out on caffeine, alcohol, sweets, fruits, vegetables, dairy, grains, or even dairy.

How do we do this? Well, it is as simple as portion control and choosing the proper ingredients for our meals. For instance, if you're having breakfast you would have:

- One store-bought, whole-wheat bagel with two tablespoons of peanut butter, without added salt of course
- 1 medium orange
- One cup of low-fat milk or lactose-free milk
- And 1 cup of decaffeinated coffee, without the sugar and cream

In the example above, not only do you have your wheat on your bagel, but you also have your protein in your peanut butter along with your coffee, dairy, and a fruit. Having this combination for breakfast will fill you up for the day while lowering your blood pressure. Each of these items is low in sodium, high in potassium, magnesium, and calcium. This breakfast gives you grains, fruit, dairy, and protein you'll need to start the day as recommended by the DASH effect diet meal plan. The best part about the DASH Effect is that you still get to have your caffeine, which helps boost your energy for the day ahead. This breakfast will provide you with the necessary nutrients that are needed to start your day on a healthy note.

The DASH effect is not like any other diet that you may have heard of. For instance, you do not have to eliminate your favorite foods. You just have to make a smarter choice when purchasing or preparing those foods. The DASH effect diet plan is so rich in potassium, magnesium, and calcium it provides a stronger foundation for your 2,000 calories nutritional intake that is recommended by the USDA for the average person. If you need a higher calorie diet, you can increase the intake of vegetables, fruits, and proteins to build a healthier balanced diet and still follow the DASH effect program.

So, "What can I eat in the DASH effect plan?" you may be asking. Well, you might be surprised to find that you can eat almost everything you already eat. It's a cleaner dietary plan with many great meal prep options that we will discuss later in this book. The DASH effect diet plan offers items such as fresh, clean, low-fat, and not processed foods. For example, you can eat fruits, vegetables, low-fat dairy, whole grains, fish, poultry, and nuts. In limited quantities, you can have beef, sweets, and sugary beverages. Caffeine and alcohol are not included in this meal plan. However, you can follow the USDA recommendation of an intake of no more than 2 alcoholic or caffeinated beverages for males per day, and no more than 1 alcoholic or caffeinated beverage for women per day. With caffeine, it is best to switch to decaffeinated beverages and eliminate the sugar and heavy cream. However, if you do have sugar in your coffee or heavy cream, you want to deduct that from your permissible caloric intake per day.

So what exactly are your permissible servings per day with the DASH effect meal plan for each food item? Let's start with your grains. You are allowed 7-8 grains per day. One serving of grains is equivalent to one slice of bread or 0.50 cup of pasta or rice. This is based on a 2,000-calorie diet per day. If you need a higher calorie intake diet, then it is suggested you do not add more grains to your servings intake, instead add more fruit or vegetables.

Your allowable vegetable servings per day are 4-5 servings. Suggested vegetables range from broccoli, carrots, tomatoes, sweet potatoes, Brussels sprouts, and other greens. A serving size is one cup of raw salad greens or a 0.50 cup of chopped vegetables. Your vegetable intake can be cooked or raw. You can use frozen or fresh vegetables. You can also have stir fry or àla carte vegetables. Adding a few extra vegetables to your meals is recommended instead of adding sweets or grains.

Fruit is another recommended dietary choice. You can have 4-5 servings of fruit per day. These servings can consist of bananas, apples, grapes, berries, and more. A medium sized fruit or 0.50 cup of fresh or frozen fruit is the suggested serving size. Fruits are a great way to have a light snack throughout the day. They also provide necessary natural sugars to your diet. Just make sure you follow the serving suggestions for snacks and meals.

Dairy is something we all struggle with. We either can't stomach it, or we drink too much heavy creams and whole milk. On the DASH effect diet plan, we can have low-fat or fat-free dairy products. These can be milk, yogurt, cheese, and other dairy items. We should have no more than 2-3 servings of dairy per day. Lactose-free products are listed within this category as well. Each serving size should be no more than one cup of milk or yogurt per serving.

If you choose to incorporate meat into your DASH food prep, then consider that you should have no more than six servings of meat per day. Each serving is 1 ounce. In most diets, we should only eat about two 3-ounce servings of meat a week. A standard deck of cards or the area of the palm of your hand is about 3 ounces of meat. It is best to have only grilled, baked, or broiled meats. Your meat choices should consist of lean ground beef, salmon, turkey, tuna, and chicken. Tuna and salmon are high in omega-3 fatty acids and helps lower cholesterol. Meat is not a required item for the DASH effect diet, so whether you add meat or not is a choice you will have to make.

Supplementing meat with legumes is perfectly fine as well. Legumes fall in the seeds category and no more than 4-5 servings per day should be consumed. These are almonds, sunflower seeds, kidney beans, peas, lentils, and other beans and nut seeds that are high in omega-3 fatty acids and monounsaturated fat. They are great to sprinkle on salads, stir-fry, and add a nice crunch to any meal. One nut to stay away from is coconuts, they do not provide the proper nutrients that you would need for this plan. A serving size for legumes is two tablespoons of sunflower seeds or 0.33 cup of nuts or beans.

You are allowed at least 2-3 servings of fats and oils per day on the DASH effect diet plan. Oils such as olive oil, margarine, and low-fat mayonnaise are all allowable oils for condiments and adding flavor. One serving size is one tablespoon of soft margarine or mayonnaise.

Although we should all avoid sweets and sugar since they add fat to our bodies, on the DASH effect diet plan there is room for five or fewer servings of sweets per week. Allowable sugars are jelly, sorbet, hard candies, and more. A serving size is one tablespoon of sugar or 0.50 cup sorbet. When adding these in try to find low-fat or fat-free options. Even low-fat cookies are a great option for you, just remember to keep track of any other ingredients that were added to the cookies like nuts.

If you are like most people, you start your day with a cup of coffee with cream and sugar. Even though these things can cause the inflammation of your body, they are allowed in the DASH effect diet plan. Men should not have more than 2 drinks per day of either coffee or alcohol, and women should have no more than 1 drink of coffee or alcohol. This is another great advantage to this dietary plan. So if you are a heavy coffee drinker, or if you love that glass of wine at night before bed, this is where the struggle might come in. By limiting the intake of these drinks, we will feel healthier, and our blood sugar will be lowered drastically as well as limit the inflammatory effects of caffeine on our body.

Why does it work?

Through extensive research and open trials conducted by the National Institute of Health, the data collected showed the patients with hypertension, high blood pressure, and diabetes experienced a decrease of symptoms while they were on the DASH effect diet plan. By gradually changing your eating habits to follow the DASH effect diet plan you are reducing your sodium intake and allowing your body to start healing. Start with one day a week and gradually work to a full week of eating healthy.

By changing your meal prep and choices for each meal, including snacks, you can gradually move up a day until you have fully integrated the DASH effect plan for every meal, seven days a week. Eliminate the sodium by not adding any more sodium to your meal prep and using an option for your foods that have a lower sodium content. A tablespoon of salt is equivalent to 2,325mg of sodium. The average person takes in 3,500mg per day. That is 1,200mg more than the standard DASH Effect plan and 2,000mg more than the lower sodium DASH plan. Preparing your meals with herbs and seasoning that have no added sodium will greatly reduce your sodium intake and aid in reducing those numbers drastically.

If your body has less sodium in it, your blood pressure drops, you start to feel better, and you can reduce your systolic blood pressure, giving you a better chance of not having a heart attack. A heart attack is one of the leading causes of death in the United States. Hypertension or high blood pressure is found in an average of 50 million people who have adhered to the American diet. That makes it about 1 billion people all over the world who are dealing with hypertension. That is why the DASH effect diet is recommended for all.

By eating foods high in potassium, magnesium, and calcium, we are lowering our blood pressure. The DASH effect is a dietary pattern, rather than a single nutrient diet, that's rich in antioxidants. It provides alternatives to junk food and eliminates the need for processed foods. By following a diet plan where you lower your sodium intake but increase your consumption of potassium, you are getting full and staying full longer allowing for fewer intakes of calories per day.

With the DASH effect diet plan, you will surely have a healthier body, and you will reduce your need for medication to control your blood pressure. It has also been shown that people who have participated in the studies exhibited signs of reduced depression. If we are happy with our health, we tend to be happier with our lives. By healing our bodies, we can heal our minds and feel like we can take on whatever life throws at us. So how do we follow this diet in our daily meal prep?

One way to follow this amazing diet plan is to ensure you have plenty of variety on the plate, you must have fruits, vegetables, and non-fat to low-fat dairy. With each meal, you should have two side dishes of vegetables and fruit-based desserts instead of desserts rich in sugar. You are eliminating the need for artificial sugars and processed foods. Reading labels before buying food helps us ensure we are buying the right ingredients and nutritional needs. We will discuss what we truly need later on in this book. For now, just know that reading labels and buying more fresh or frozen food options is our best way to ensure we are following the recommended food list.

In a typical DASH Effect daily meal plan, our nutritional values can look like this:

- Calories 2015
- Total fat 70g
- Saturated fat 10g
- Trans fat 0g
- Monounsaturated fat 25g
- Potassium 3,274mg
- Calcium 1,298mg
- Cholesterol 70 mg
- Sodium 1,607mg
- Total Carbohydrates 267g
- Dietary fiber 39g
- Total sugar 109g
- Protein 90g

- Magnesium 394mg

As you can see, the amount of sodium, sugar, saturated fat, and trans fat is reduced while the amount of potassium, magnesium, and calcium is increased, providing a better diet rich in nutrients. This is how we can lower our blood pressure, decrease our blood sugar, enhance the functions of our kidney, so we can feel healthier, alert, and energized.

Chapter 2: The Key Concepts Behind the DASH Effect

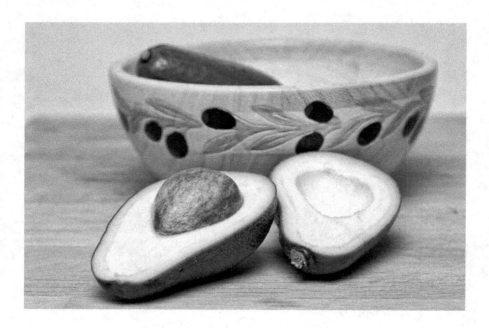

The DASH effect diet is a therapeutic approach to eating healthier. It helps you manage your weight, your blood pressure, your insulin sensitivity, and your blood cholesterol. What really makes the DASH effect diet great is that it not only lowers the blood pressure but it also, over time, helps you reduce your reliance on chemical substances. It is recommended for everyone from children to seniors who are trying to live healthy as much as possible. Not only does it provide health benefits, but it also has added benefit of helping you lose weight. There are no expensive supplements or shakes to purchase, making it a budget-friendly option for people who have limited funds. By eliminating processed foods, high sodium foods, all the fat in dairy, and lowering your intake of red meats, it also provides you with a low-sodium meal plan that will drastically reduce your risks of being afflicted with heart disease and cancer as well as diabetes and depression.

As with any diet or meal prep plan, there are key factors that determine why we need to change our eating habits. Whether it is high blood pressure or finding a healthier weight loss program, changing your dietary intake is hard. We don't make decisions to change our eating habits because we are told to by our doctors, it's not because the hottest stars are doing it, and it's not because we see our best friend or others online getting healthier either. It's because you are dealing with illness and want a better way to handle it, it is because you are ready to change your life and health.

When you get to the point that you have had enough of the pain, enough of the suffering from high blood pressure, enough of multiple prescriptions and are ready to make a difference in your life and your family's lives, that is when we start thinking about changing. By adding the DASH effect diet to our meal prep plans, we can start making those changes with minimal discomfort or inconvenience.

One thing we must be prepared to do is accepting that we no longer need the sodium and that food will taste good without it. Just give it time. After you eliminate all the sodium you have been adding to your meals, you will start to feel better, and your health will improve. You will notice that the taste of food has changed, and you will be able to taste more of the food and less of the sodium. Once you start the elimination process, you may feel as if your food has lost its flavor, but it hasn't. That is just the sodium leaving your body. Your taste buds will adjust themselves. Over time, you will start to taste the food, and you will have a deeper understanding of how your food should taste. You will have less of a craving for sodium, and you will even be able to tell if extra sodium was added to your food.

The key factor to making this change, and sticking with it, is to gradually reduce your sodium. Start with buying foods with low-sodium content and only sprinkling salt on the food while it cooks. Use a specific measurement and don't add any more after it is done. Gradually eliminate this habit of sprinkling salt and get used to the natural sodium that's in your food. As you decrease your sodium intake, you will notice your taste buds adjusting, and you will no longer need the sodium that you used to put on your food. The same goes for sugar and other things that you need to adjust to this diet.

By adding more fruit and vegetables to your meals, you are essentially getting those natural sugars that are necessary for your dietary and nutritional needs. Everything we eat has natural sugars, as young children we learn that sugar is good. However, we are not told that sugar can be found naturally in fruits and vegetables. As we get older, we struggle to let go of the sugars that we have added to our diet. Those sugars cause fat to build up in our bodies and can result in a higher risk of diabetes. Salt and sugar are among the hardest things to let go of, but it can happen.

If we eat healthier, we become healthier and more energized. Sugar and salt weigh us down and even make us look bloated. This can make us less energized and uncomfortable in our clothes. It increases our heart rate and changes the chemistry in our bodies. When we become healthier, our moods change, we can think better, and we won't have as many health issues. These are the key concepts behind the DASH effect diet plan.

Dietary recommendations with nutritional facts

A few dietary recommendations can make a world of difference as we transition to a new meal prep plan. What you should start with is some general knowledge about what nutrients are found in our foods. For example, fruits are low fast-food items with low sodium and lower cholesterol. This makes them a great source of vitamin C, folic acid, and dietary fiber. Fruits that are high in potassium are bananas, cantaloupe, dried apricots, and orange juice. Dietary fiber is found in fruits and can help reduce heart disease and helps with fiber intake which aids in bowel functions. Whole fruits contain enough dietary fiber to make you feel full, so you will only require a minimum amount of calories. Vitamin C helps repair body tissue and is necessary to maintain healthy teeth and gums.

Several vegetables have zero sodium content. Asparagus is one of these vegetables. If you add 5 spears of asparagus to a meal, that's enough to significantly reduce your sodium intake. Other zero-sodium vegetables are ⅓ portion of a medium cucumber, ¾ cups of green snap peas, ½ medium summer squash and 1 medium sweet corn ear. Try incorporating these into your meal prep plans. Every meal should have 1-2 vegetables. So think about adding in several more choices to your dinner plate.

Tilapia, tuna, salmon, catfish, and halibut all have low-sodium content. With a serving size of 3 ounces, you can incorporate either one of these fish into just about every meal. For example, you can have poached salmon and eggs for breakfast. Add in a cup of decaffeinated coffee and a slice of whole-wheat bread with light margarine and a medium apple, and you have yourself a very hearty breakfast with low sodium and a minimal number of processed foods. In this chapter, I have included several recipes and nutritional facts to help you start the DASH effect diet on your own.

The dietary needs of everyone and every age is different so following the standard 2000 calorie diet may not be the ideal diet plan for everyone. So I have included a dietary recommendation for women and men based on age groups below.

Age (Women)	Sedentary lifestyle	Moderate lifestyle	Active lifestyle
19-30	2000	2000-2200	2400
31-50	1800	2000	2200
51+	1600	1800	2000-2200
Age (Men)			
19-30	2400	2600-2800	3000
31-50	2200	2400-2600	2800-3000
51+	2000	2200-2400	2400-2800

Using these dietary daily nutritional values, we can then design a meal plan that incorporates these needs into the total calorie intake for the day. Below are a few recipes for meal prep items that can be used with fruit, grain, low-fat dairy, meat, and nuts or seeds of your choice. I started with a couple of breakfast recipes then provided you with a couple of lunch recipes as well as a couple of dinner recipes. Each recipe is designed to follow the DASH effect diet and is just a piece of the menu. You will notice that I have included alternatives to traditional flour as well as a vegan alternative for those who do not eat meats. Each recipe also indicates the nutritional value. Some of these recipes provide recommended toppings or garnish, and some of them are great to bring along to work as a snack or lunch.

Recipes for breakfast

Banana Pancakes

If you love bananas, then you are going to love these pancakes. This recipe should make about 4-6 pancakes and takes roughly 30-40 minutes to prepare.

Nutrition per serving:

- Calories 146
- Fat 4g
- Carbohydrates 22g
- Protein 7g
- Sodium 331g

What to use:

- Low-fat milk or lactose-free milk (0.33 cup)

- Chopped walnuts (1 tablespoon)

- Vanilla extract (0.50 teaspoon)

- Olive oil (1.50 teaspoon)

- Cinnamon (A small pinch)

- Salt (A small pinch)

- Large Eggs (2)

- Baking powder (1.0 teaspoon)

- Whole-wheat flour or coconut flour (0.33 cup)

- Mashed Banana (1)

What to do:

1. In a mixing bowl, combine all of the dry ingredients.
2. Separate the two eggs but keep the egg whites
3. In another mixing bowl, add olive oil, low-fat milk, egg whites, mashed banana, and vanilla until it's blended together well.
4. Combine the dry ingredients with the liquid ingredients. Using a spoon, stir until it's smooth.
5. Heat a griddle or frying pan over medium heat and apply a lite coating of olive oil to prevent the mixture from sticking. Place ¼ cup of the pancake mixture into a pan.
6. When you see bubbles around the edges of the pancakes, flip them over and continue cooking until the other side is done.
7. Sprinkle the chopped walnuts on top for added protein and texture.

Toppings:

- Sugar-free syrup
- Non-fat vanilla yogurt

Homemade Granola

This recipe takes 10 minutes to prepare, 30 minutes to cook, and makes 16 servings.

Nutrition per serving:

- Calories 199
- Fat 13g
- Sodium 86mg
- Carbohydrates 16g
- Protein 5g

What to use:

- Olive oil or Coconut oil (0.33 cup)
- Honey or Maple Syrup (0.33 cup)
- Salt (0.50 teaspoon)
- Cinnamon (2 Teaspoons)
- Protein Powder (0.50 cup)
- Flaxseed meal (0.50 cup)
- Raw pumpkin seeds (0.50 cup)
- Chopped walnuts (1 cup)
- Oats (2 cups)

What to do:

1. Start with preheating your oven to 325 °F.

2. Combine oats, walnuts, pumpkin seeds, flax, protein powder, cinnamon, and salt in a large mixing bowl.

3. Once everything is mixed well, drizzle with honey and then olive oil.

4. Stir until the mixture is evenly coated with both.

5. Prepare a baking sheet with wax paper.

6. Spread the mixture over the wax paper.

7. Continue to bake at 325°F for 30 minutes until golden brown.

8. Once done remove the granola from the stove and let it cool in the fridge for 2 hours.

Recipes for lunch

Spicy Peanut Tofu, Rice, and Avocado Salad

This recipe needs about 15 minutes to prepare. Serving size of 2 entrée sized salads.

Nutrition per serving:

- Calories 380 kcal
- Fat 18g

- Carbohydrates 42g

- Protein 15g

- Iron 14%

- Calcium 16%

- Vitamin A 15%

- Vitamin C 12%

What to use:

Dressing:

- Cayenne pepper (3-4 Dashes)

- Tamari (2 teaspoons)

- Water (0.50 cup)

- Agave syrup or Maple syrup (2 teaspoons)

- White miso paste (1 tablespoon)

- Peanut butter (2 tablespoons)

Salad:

- Mixed Spring greens (5 cups)

- Avocado, sliced-lengthwise (0.50 cups)

- Firm tofu, chilled and cubed (0.50 cup)

- Cooked brown rice (1 cup)

Garnish:

- Chopped cilantro

- Chopped peanuts

- Pepper or cayenne sprinkled on top (dash)

What to do:

1. Prepare your food processor or Vitamix.
2. Combine all the ingredients for the dressing in the food processor or Vitamix.
3. Blend until it's smooth and adjust the peanut butter as needed to get the richness of the sauce you wish for.
4. Prepare a pot with water and a pinch of salt. Once boiled, add the rice.
5. Cook rice until tender and done.
6. On a cutting board, dice up your tofu.
7. Toss your tofu in with the rice.
8. Add in a few spoonfuls of peanut sauce then proceed to toss the salad.
9. Place greens in a serving bowl.
10. Place sliced avocado over the top of the greens.
11. Decorating in a twirl design.
12. Place a scoop of the peanut tofu on top of the salad.
13. Add more dressing as needed, plus the cilantro and peanuts, cayenne pepper.

Poppy Seed Chicken Noodle Casserole

This is a twist on the classic chicken casserole. It takes 50 minutes to bake chicken and up to 2 hours once it's placed in the slow cooker. Serving size is 4.

Nutrition per serving:

- Calories 411.3
- Total Fat 8.1 g
- Cholesterol 68.4 mg
- Sodium 251.8 mg
- Carbohydrates 47.4 g
- Protein 38.7 g

What to use:

- Light buttery spread (4 tablespoons)
- Poppy seed (2 Teaspoons)
- Frozen peas (2 cups Thawed)
- Whole-wheat pasta (4 cups)
- Boneless and skinless chicken breast (2)

What to do:

1. Preheat oven to 325 °F.
2. Once it's preheated, place the chicken in a pan and cook.

3. While cooking chicken, cook the pasta until it's tender.

4. Once the pasta is done, place it in the slow cooker on low temperature.

5. Add the peas.

6. Add the poppy seeds.

7. Add the buttery spread.

8. Once the chicken is done, add it too.

9. Cook in the slow cooker until the peas are warm or for 30 minutes minimum or 2 hours maximum.

10. Season to taste.

Recipes for dinner

Easy Sweet Potato Veggie Burgers, with Avocado

This is a vegan twist on the traditional burger. Who says burgers can't be vegan?

This recipe makes 6-8 burgers and takes 10 minutes to prepare and 80 minutes to cook.

Nutrition per serving:

- Total carbohydrates: 30g
- Protein: 7g
- Fat: 4g
- Calories: 176g
- Dietary fiber: 5g

THE SIMPLE KETOGENIC DIET

What to use:

- Chopped greens (kale, spinach, parsley) (0.33-1 cup finely)
- Nutritional yeast or any flour (try oat flour) (0.33 cup)
- Black pepper (add more for more bite!) (0.25 teaspoon)
- Salt (0.50 teaspoon)
- Chipotle powder or Cajun spice (use more for spicier burgers, (0.50 -1 teaspoon)
- Garlic powder (1 teaspoon)
- Apple cider vinegar (0.75 teaspoon)
- Tahini (2-3 tablespoons)
- White onion, chopped (0.50 cup)
- Cooked white beans (canned, drained and rinsed) (16 ounces)
- Sweet potato, baked and peeled (1 medium)

Toppings:

- Avocado, tomato, Vegenaise, burger buns, greens

Skillet:

- Virgin coconut oil (1 tablespoon)

Optional:

- Panko breadcrumbs for crispy coating

What to do:

1. Preheat oven to 400 °F.

2. Bake the potato for 40-60 minutes or until tender.

3. Combine potato and beans in a large mixing bowl. Beans must be rinsed before you add it to the bowl.

4. Using fork or masher, mash together the ingredients in the bowl.

5. Put in the white onions and keep mashing.

6. Put in the tahini, garlic, chipotle, salt and pepper, yeast, greens, and apple cider vinegar.

7. Keep on mashing until it's thoroughly mashed.

8. With the oven at 400 °F, heat a skillet on the stovetop over high heat and add the coconut oil.

9. Form burger patties and roll in panko crumbs if using them then place on the skillet to cook.

10. Cooking time is 1-3 minutes per side, cook patties until light brown.

11. Then repeat with all the rest of the patties, making around 6-8 patties.

12. Once all the patties are cooked, place them on a baking sheet lined with wax paper and bake for 10-15 minutes, cooking all the way through.

13. While baking the burgers, slice up your toppings for decorating the burgers.

14. Toast your whole-wheat bun in a toaster (any whole-wheat, high-fiber bun will work).

15. Add vegan mayonnaise and spicy mustard to the bun

16. When burgers are done add burger to bun and the top with your choice of toppings.

17. Serve warm!

Note: You can store the remaining burgers in a sealed container in the fridge for a day or freezer for a week. You just have to reheat it at 400 °F for about 12 minutes.

Easy Roasted Salmon

This is part of a dinner dish that includes roasted salmon. Also, you will add vegetables and fruit along with some grain. This recipe takes 10 minutes to prepare and 22 minutes to cook. Serving size of 4.

Nutrition per serving:

- Sodium 78 mg
- Calories 251
- Potassium 894 mg
- Calcium 36 mg
- Cholesterol 94 mg
- Carbohydrates 2 g
- Fat 11g
- Magnesium 53 mg
- Saturated Fat 2g
- Dietary Fiber less than 1 g
- Sugars less than 1 g
- Protein 34g

THE SIMPLE KETOGENIC DIET

What to use:

- Garlic cloves, minced and peeled (4)

- Fresh ground pepper

- Lemon, cut (4 wedges)

- Minced fresh dill, from one small bunch (0.25 cup)

- Wild salmon fillets (4-6 ounce pieces)

What to do:

1. Preheat oven to 400 °F before starting.

2. Bring out a glass baking dish and coat it with coconut oil.

3. Place your salmon fillets in the dish.

4. Using the 4 wedges of lemon, squeeze one per fillet on top of the fillets.

5. Then sprinkle black pepper, garlic, and dill on each fillet.

6. Bake for 20-22 minutes until the fillets are opaque in the center.

Chocolate Banana Cake

This is a blend of chocolate and banana which blends really well with the cake texture. The preparation time is about 15 minutes and cooking time is around 25 minutes. This recipe can make around 18 servings.

Nutrition per serving:

- Calories: 150
- Sodium: 52 milligrams
- Potassium: 119 milligrams
- Magnesium: 19 milligrams

What to use:

- Large egg (1)
- Canola oil (0.25 cup)
- Soy milk (0.75 cup)
- Ripe banana, mashed (1 large, 0.50 cup)
- Baking soda (0.50 teaspoon)
- Splenda brown sugar blend (0.50 cup)
- Unsweetened cocoa powder (0.25 cup)
- Semisweet dark chocolate chips (0.50 cup)
- All-purpose flour (2 cups)
- Vanilla extract (1 teaspoon)
- Egg white (1)
- Lemon juice (1 tablespoon)

What to do:

1. Preheat your oven to 350 °F.
2. Using olive oil, coat a nonstick brownie pan.
3. Add flour to a bowl.
4. Blend in the brown sugar.
5. Cocoa and baking soda.
6. In a separate bowl throw in the bananas.
7. While whisking, pour in the soy milk, oil, eggs, egg whites, lemon juice, and the vanilla.
8. Once everything is blended, make a cavity in the flour and slowly pour in the liquid mix.
9. Add the chocolate chips.
10. Using a wooden spoon, stir to blend the ingredients.
11. Once it's thoroughly blended, spoon mixture into a brownie pan.
12. Bake for 25 minutes.
13. Take it out and use a toothpick to check the center if it is cooked all the way through.

Chapter 3: Why We Need the DASH Effect to Stay in Peak Form

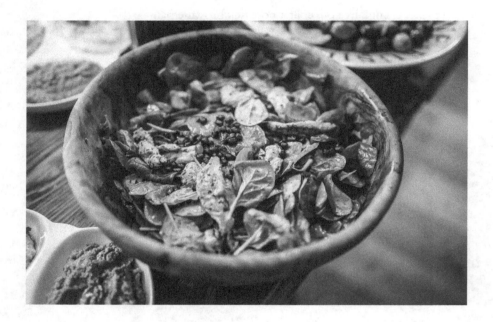

Now that you know a little bit more about the DASH effect diet and how it helps your body become healthier, let's discuss why you need the DASH effect and how the myths and negative misconceptions should not be an issue once you're on this meal plan.

As we grow up, our diets get discombobulated, and we start consuming too many fried foods, too much fat, heavy creams, and way more sugar and sodium than we should have ever consumed. There is no clear-cut reason why we do this. As we age, we start trying new things, and we find an easier way to prepare meals, and we all too often take the lazy choice of stopping at the local McDonald's. Through years of eating unhealthy foods, we developed high blood pressure, insulin spikes, heart conditions, diabetes, and even depression.

We don't consider that our diet is the main cause, so we go to the doctor and get medicine that is designed with chemicals, similar to the processed foods that we have been consuming for years. The medicines help, but they do not eliminate the problem, in fact, they increase our need to be dependent on chemical-based foods and medicine. So what do we do about it? We continue to eat the garbage that is killing us, and we wonder why we aren't getting any better.

This is a cycle of self-destruction that we have carried from the early stages of life where we learned our eating habits and developed a taste for food. The DASH effect diet is against what we know as the normal way to enjoy our foods. It scares people to think that lower sodium could actually transform their health. If you are anything like the average American, you probably didn't realize the amount of sodium that is in your standard everyday diet.

That is why the DASH effect diet is the ideal way to get your health back on track. We don't need added salt in our foods. We don't need to consume 66 pounds of sugar per year. We definitely don't need to be dependent on chemical-based food and drinks. So how do we change this? We follow the DASH effect diet.

If you have been following me up until now, then you know that there are many benefits you can gain from following the DASH effect diet, and you are probably considering changing your eating habits. Maybe you're a little hesitant about eliminating the sugar and salt in your diet. You probably think that your food will not taste as good. Maybe you have tried other diets in the past, but you always ended up falling back on your old eating patterns.

Well, the good thing about the DASH effect diet is that it isn't like any other diet on the market. That is because it isn't a diet plan at all. It is a complete change in your eating patterns. But you don't have to actually change much of what you are already doing. It's mostly about portion control and buying cleaner and fresher ingredients.

If you are part of the meat-eating community that consumes 52.2 million pounds of meat per year, then it may be a bit difficult to alter your meat options for a while. In the DASH effect plan, you eat less red meat and more poultry, fish, and turkey. These are leaner meats with less fat and cholesterol. They also have a lower sodium content than pork and beef. If you are not a meat eater, then this diet will be an easy change for you. Many of the recipes that are available on the DASH effect diet are not only dairy-free but meat-free as well, making this a vegan-friendly diet.

Every year more and more people are being diagnosed with hypertension, diabetes, and heart disease. With the alarming numbers of people who suffer with these disorders, we need to consider why no one has changed their diet plan. Maybe it is out of fear of losing control over their food options. Maybe it is just because of plain stubborn behavior. Whatever the reason may be, Americans are not changing their eating patterns, it is clear that continuing the cycle of fat, deep fried, high-sodium meals are not doing any wonders for their health. The DASH effect is recommended not only by one scientist but by several companies and agencies who fight for a healthier America.

Why should you transition to the DASH effect diet? The answer: because it simply works. It's that simple and that easy. Scientifically, it has been proven to work. If something works as well as this does, it's a surprise that the school systems are not incorporating it into their weekly meal prepping for students.

How the benefits outweigh any myths or negative press on the effects

So why hasn't it taken off? There is a long-running myth that fresh foods are not as cheap as processed foods. But this simply isn't true. The process of preparing fresher foods that are richer in vitamins and nutrients and contain less fat-burning calories means that you will need a lower intake of calories and that your food will keep you full longer, essentially costing less in the long run.

People often believe that going to the drive-thru at McDonald's or Burger King is easier than preparing a kale salad. After a long day at work, you don't feel like coming home to prepare a healthy meal. It takes longer, and you just don't have the time or energy. This too is not true. It takes about 15 minutes to prepare a meal acceptable for the DASH effect diet, once all the prep work has been completed. You can also prepackage your ingredients or practice food prep procedures by preparing your ingredients before work and placing them in a slow cooker to simmer all day. This allows for you to simply come home, grab a bowl, and relax on the couch or at the table with family while enjoying a healthy, clean, and fresh meal.

Many people believe that there is a learning curve to proper nutritional calorie intake food prep. This as well is not true. There are so many recipes and cookbooks on the market that are geared towards healthier and cleaner eating that you'll find a recipe in no time to prepare for dinner. The best part is whatever you have left over from dinner can be utilized for breakfast or even lunch depending on what it is. Many of our food options on the DASH effect diet plan can be used for multiple meals, such as apples can be used as breakfast, fruit side dishes, and even desserts.

Often times, people think that eating healthy means eating bland food. That simply isn't true. Just because it's healthy doesn't make it bland. There are so many reasons why this myth is present, one of them being that throughout our life we have added salt and sugar to everything we eat, chose the fattest parts of the meat, and excessively flavored our foods. We do this because we are conditioned into thinking that we must add flavor to food. However, food already has a flavor. The natural juices and flavors that are ingrained in the fruit and vegetables provide all the flavor you need for your meal to taste amazing.

Now that doesn't mean that adding herbs to your food isn't a good thing. Many herbs and nectars provide healing benefits that just can't be ignored. Rosemary helps with immunity and honey is an antihistamine. Garlic is good for reducing blood pressure as well as combating the common cold. Sage is known for its anti-inflammatory properties as well as antioxidants. As you can see, many herbs and nectars provide added benefits to your food. So the best rule of thumb is to taste the natural foods then add in a few flavors through fresh herbs to give it an added health benefit.

Herbs can be purchased dried as well as fresh. Many people believe the benefits of herbs are just as effective when dried. I find that fresh herbs give a much better aromatic smell and tend to have a fresher, cleaner taste. They blend better with our foods and gives that added touch of texture that you just can't get from powders or dried herbs. They also are not processed heavily and have not been mixed with added sodium and other chemicals to make them last longer. As with any fresh food, being frozen is the best route since they still retain all the nutrients that provide you with the healthiest caloric intake.

Many Americans have been buying processed and canned foods since World War 2. They are marketed as containing all the health benefits of a fresh batch of vegetables. However, through the process of canning or processing at the factory, we have learned that they are missing key components to their nutritional value. So the myth that canned or processed foods are just as good as fresh is completely wrong. Not only are they higher in sodium, since it is added for flavor and sustainability. But they are having their key nutrients flash steamed or cooked out of them and then being mixed with sustainable chemicals to make them last longer on the shelf. Taking all this into account, we should always purchase our foods frozen or fresh to ensure we are feeding ourselves and our families the best possible combination of nutrients that we can afford. One way we can do this is through farmers' markets and at local farms.

Buying your food at a farmers' market or picking your own at a local farm can also reduce the cost of the food you are purchasing. Knowing what you want to prepare in advance is also a way of reducing your cost of groceries, and it will also provide you with a guideline to decide on what kind of meal you should cook each day. This allows you to prepare your ingredients in advance and be ready for mealtime without the extra hassle. It doesn't take a ton of extra time to learn how to prepare in advance. You simply need to know what you like and have a recipe or idea of how you want to prepare a meal once you're ready for meal prep time. This will cut down on the amount of time it takes to prepare the meal without adding extra time to your daily to-do list. Later in this book, we will lay out a method to meal prep with a list of options for each meal and a way to incorporate an accountability partner into your diet change.

Chapter 4: Who Should Not Use the DASH Effect and Why?

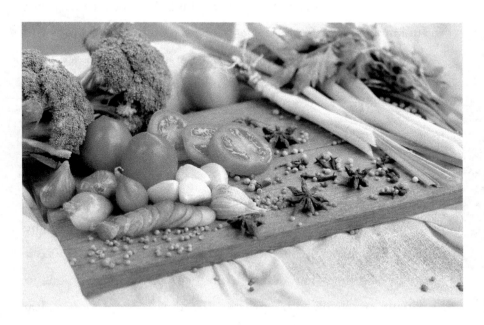

Previously, we discussed who the DASH Effect diet is ideal for. As rated by the Food and Drug Administration the DASH Effect diet is rated safe for everyone. So who shouldn't use the DASH effect diet then? Well, that is simple, this diet is not for people that are not committed to making a positive change in their lives. If you do not want to be healthier, if you do not want to lose weight, if you enjoy having diabetes and hypertension, if you do not want to transform your health and make changes to your lifestyle that will reduce your blood pressure, help you lose weight and also feel more happy in general about life, then you should not use the DASH effect diet.

Who in your family does this sound like? Is this person you? Or is it someone else that has been using their disease as a reason to play the victim every day of their life? You see the DASH effect diet is not for quitters. It's not for those people who love having sickness and struggle to keep up with their children or grandchildren. It is not for those that would rather eat a high-sodium and high-sugar diet. It is definitely not for those people who think that if their food is not loaded with bacon grease, it's not good.

In today's families, we all have that one person that doesn't watch what they eat. They think food doesn't determine their health, or they just really don't care. That person is not the ideal person to try the DASH effect diet. Not because they don't need it, not because it wouldn't help them, and definitely not because they are immune to its benefits or allergic to the process. No, those people are not ideal for the DASH effect diet because they do not care how they are treating their bodies. They don't care if they have ailments that they can reduce and eliminate. The simply do not care about the state of their health.

So how do you help those who don't care? We all would know they need the DASH effect diet and that if they were to give it a try, they would not only be happier, but they will also see drastic changes in their health for the better. So instead of shoving the DASH effect diet down their throats and trying to force them to get healthy, we must first get healthy ourselves. The best way to lead someone to a better path for their life is to show them through your own actions that it works and to essentially trigger their jealousy, so they want to get healthy to spite you.

Now I know this sounds a bit petty and far-fetched, but isn't it true that sometimes you only wanted something simply because someone else had it? Exactly, so now you see where this chapter is going. So far we have discussed what the DASH effect diet is, whom it's suited for, why it is effective, and now we will discuss the positive effects it has on our mental psyche.

Have you ever done something that you thought you were going to fail at, but in the end you actually did not fail? What about winning an award for something you did inadvertently while doing something else? Well, that feeling you got when that award was won, or that amazing realization that you actually succeeded instead of failing is what the DASH effect diet does for your psyche. Imagine going in for a haircut and coming out with a stylish haircut, a new dye job, and some free hair-conditioning supplies.

When you get so focused on creating a healthy eating habit you forget about so many other things that you are accomplishing. Such as losing weight or lowering your insulin injection needs. What if we could all just wake up with no depression, no diseases, no cancers, and no excess fat? With the DASH effect diet, we eventually can. Now, do you still want to question the validity of the DASH effects?

To get healthy and reduce your blood pressure you have to start somewhere, and the DASH effect diet is exactly where you need to start. Do not be disappointed if you have setbacks because they are normal. As long as you figure out the triggers and do what you can to avoid them you should be able to continue the program without too many setbacks.

But what if my blood pressure isn't elevated? Well, then the DASH effect diet is still the best for you. It is a starting point for a healthier and cleaner lifestyle. No, I don't mean cleaner like you cleaned your house. By saying cleaner, I mean that your food comes from the ground, with no pesticides, no growth hormones, no chemicals, and no processing.

What else do you need to know to understand that the DASH effect diet is for everyone? All it takes to find out if it is for you, besides me telling you it is, is to get started today. In this book, I have provided you a detailed description of what the DASH effect is and how to incorporate it into your life. But one thing we haven't talked about yet is the motivation you need to bring about changes in your life with the DASH effect. That is what this whole chapter will be on, motivational techniques to keep you focused, to keep you moving forward, and to show those stubborn family members who think that food does not heal, that in fact, it does.

One proven method to motivate you to continue on your journey with the DASH effect diet is to see progress. Progress is wonderful. It's like a reward in itself. When you see that your blood pressure is lower or you are experiencing less blood sugar spikes for example. That is called progress. Maybe your doctor has noticed a positive change in your blood. Maybe when you stand in front of the mirror after your shower, you see a slimmer and healthier you. Progress can be anything from a slight change in the size of your pants to a drastic drop in your need for your blood pressure medication. Whatever progress you achieved, regardless of how small it is, you need to celebrate.

Celebrate in ways that don't undermine your progress. There are many ways to celebrate your progress without having to derail your new lifestyle. One of my favorite ways to celebrate a positive change in my life is to immediately give myself praise. I look myself in the mirror, and I tell myself all the things that are wonderful about what I have accomplished. I acknowledge the efforts I have made, and I congratulate myself on a job well done. This is a personalized pat on the back.

Another way to reward yourself is to buy yourself a new piece of clothing, something that fits your new waistline. This tells your mind that you are making changes to get a more beneficial lifestyle. It also gives you a wonderful endorphin boost when you look at that new, slim piece of clothing and think, "I did this." Just remember that you are working towards a healthier you and that healthier 'you' will need a whole new wardrobe eventually. By throwing away clothes that no longer fit, you are subconsciously telling your mind and body that you will no longer accept what your body was back then. This is like a confirmation that you are a new person. Buying new clothes helps us physically see the changes we are making, giving us a good reason to celebrate our accomplishments and progress while making sure we look amazing.

Accountability is another great way to reward yourself when you see great progress. Accountability is when someone else will hold you accountable for your goals. This will be discussed later in Chapter 6, but for now, we will just state that accountability is calling your friend, your mom, or your exercise buddy and celebrating with them about your progress. Remember they are on your side and know that you need this healthier lifestyle.

There are so many ways to celebrate your achievements. By setting goals and reaching them, you are rewarding yourself every day when you pick healthier options and become a healthier you. Sometimes just knowing is enough of a reward. However, if knowing that you are getting healthier isn't enough, you can always try a day at the spa, a movie with your best friend, or even a night out with your favorite girl/guy.

One of the best rewards you can give yourself is acknowledging that you have done it on your own, without medicines, without surgeries, and without sitting around thinking there is nothing you can do to get healthier. You are the deciding factor, and you made that one decision to make your life better. Whatever you choose as a reward, make sure it is something that will give you excitement and that feeling of accomplishment. When we don't feel like we accomplished something big, we tend to feel more sad than happy. The trick is to be excited about your progress even if it seems insignificant.

Chapter 5: Specific Benefits to Your Health Gained from the DASH Effect

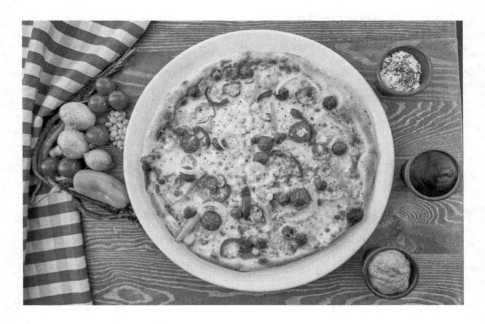

Since you made it this far, you have heard over and over that the DASH effect has outstanding scientific evidence showing its validity and the effects it has on your health. So what more can I say to motivate you on getting started with the DASH effect diet? Maybe with the amazing effects the DASH diet can have on our health, we will see a potential for lower insurance rates. Not only are our insurance rates on the verge of dropping because of this amazing diet, but it's also a national dietary method that's been recommended for over 10 years. Another benefit to the DASH effect diet is that previous studies proved that staying on the DASH effect diet can result in a reduction of systolic and diastolic blood pressure. These results were across all age groups, races, and genders. That means that this diet works for all races.

We all know that many African Americans suffer from race-specific anomalies and that these anomalies can cause certain diseases to be more dominant and prevalent. One thing scientists learned in the trials was that this diet worked amazingly on the African American community as well as the Caucasians, Asians, and Indians.

Further findings revealed that the DASH effect diet also lowered the risk of stroke and coronary heart disease, making it beneficial for people who are afflicted with such conditions. The DASH effect diet has also helped with bone loss and density, reducing bone turnover, which means an improvement in bone health for those prone to osteoporosis.

There are many ways for the DASH effect diet to help you with weight loss. Below are just a few of the ways:

- Fruits and veggies are low in calories.
- They are more filling as well
- You include protein-rich foods in every meal
- Using protein for snacks can increase your energy
- Protein makes meals more satisfying
- Protein also helps with in-between blood sugar crashes

- By focusing on the healthy foods, you eliminate the need for junk foods
- By eating denser foods, you reduce your cravings
- You can make the DASH effect diet your lifestyle diet plan
- It's not a fad diet
- Carbohydrates are not used to fill you up
- The plan doesn't limit your protein
- There is less starch
- Protein supports muscle mass
- Proteins are energy boosters and provide us the energy to exercise more efficiently

High blood pressure is a big reason why the DASH effect is popular. By reducing your sodium intake, you end up reducing your blood pressure. There are a few other benefits that we haven't discussed throughout this book:

- It helps reduce your blood pressure by reducing sodium in your diet
- It also helps by reducing your weight which can raise your blood pressure
- By reducing your weight and raising your protein intake you have more energy
- More energy means you can exercise more and help lower your blood pressure
- The DASH effect diet provides a healthy eating plan that not only reduces your blood pressure but helps keep it stabilized

We all know that high blood pressure increases the risk of getting heart disease and can contribute to several other diseases and ailments. The DASH effect can help eliminate the chances of heart disease by lowering your blood pressure. Several of the benefits of the DASH effect have been discussed throughout this book and in this chapter. But there are more benefits that the DASH effect can provide to aid in lowering the risk of heart disease:

- By adding more fiber, calcium, and magnesium, you can reduce the risk of heart disease
- Those three minerals help regulate blood pressure
- Potassium stops the effects of sodium
- The DASH effect diet is a sustainable diet, it is not something that will end immediately
- It's low in sodium and high in nutrient-rich foods
- It is adaptable, low stress, and easily customizable, making it the best diet choice for all

Even with all the benefits that the DASH effect diet has been proven to have on your health, not many people are using it. Though it has changed the way people think about eating and how food can transform your health, people are still so reluctant to what they have considered as proper eating their whole life. So why are more people not using the DASH effect diet? This is partly because the patients who need the diet the most are only getting medicinal help from their primary care providers. Not many doctors have nutritional backgrounds and lack knowledge in this area. Perhaps many people can be helped immensely if part of a doctor's training included nutrition and diet plans.

Although doctors are not trained to properly help those dealing with a diet issue, nutritionists are, and there are many ways you can get in contact with one. Health coaches are trained to help you find the right diet plan for your needs. Some of them should be listed in your local online business directory. Finding the right coach to help you with the DASH effect diet will take some time. Try asking family and friends. Get opinions online from trusted friends. Research the options in your area and know exactly what you are looking for.

Even with all the research and referrals, you still won't be able to know if that coach is right for you until you have a face-to-face meeting with them. So sit down with the coach of your choice and ask all the questions that you need to. Make sure you make a list of the questions you want to ask, this will ensure that you will get to know that person better. Once you run out of questions, ask the coach if there is anything else they would like to include in their comments or if they have any questions. This is a sure way to hear out your coach's opinions.

Remember they are the experts and know exactly what to do to help you with your dietary needs. One question you might ask is: "Are they familiar with the DASH effect diet?" This should instantly tell you whether or not they are the right nutritionist for you.

With all the talk about nutrition, food portions, and benefits associated with the DASH effect diet, this book would not be complete without helpful tools. These tools are designed to teach you how to incorporate proper meal preparations, exercise, accountability, and so much more. For the next chapter, we will be looking at those tools, and we will learn how to utilize them. The first tool we will look at is accountability, how you can find an accountability partner, and what you can expect from an accountability partner. You will notice that in this section we discussed nutritionists and health coaches a little bit more. That is because a health coach is a great accountability partner. Part of their roles in your life is to help you become accountable for your food choices, they act as your support system, and of course, they're your motivational coach.

The next part would deal with the subject of getting healthy with the help of exercise. We discussed various ways to incorporate exercise into your healthy lifestyle. There are many forms of exercise, and as a person with health issues, you might want to consult a doctor about appropriate exercises that you can do without endangering your health. Making sure that you are not overexerting yourself or injuring yourself is the best way to start a new exercise routine. In the next chapter, we will talk about yoga, running, jogging, and cardio. These are all acceptable exercises even for someone who has been dealing with various health concerns.

Meal prep is a big part of the DASH effect diet, and it can make or break your progress. Since you were proactive and bought this book, you have already set yourself up for success. This book not only explains the information on why this diet plan works, but it also helps you prepare the right meals so that you can take complete advantage of the DASH effect diet. Meal preparation is an easy thing to do if you use the worksheet provided in the next chapter. There is a designated section for each day and each meal. There is also a list of serving sizes and approved foods.

This is just a starting point. Once you get the hang of the process, you will find yourself creating your own meal preparation worksheets or even designing a digital one to use on the go. Meal preparation sounds like a chore, but you shouldn't feel discouraged because it can give you something to look forward to, such as that amazing meal you planned for the next day.

But meal preparations would be nothing without the calorie intake worksheet. It is designed to show you during the first few weeks of your journey into the DASH effect diet how well you are following the guidelines set by the program. By keeping track of the calories that you are taking in and making sure you stay within the recommended limits for each nutrient, you are following the program as designed. Doing what you can to meet the requirements of the DASH effect diet can help make sure that you will arrive at the desired outcome, a healthier and happier life.

Chapter 6: Ways to Include the DASH Effect into Your Daily Meals

There is so much information about the DASH effect diet packed into this book that I'm sure it is confusing, and you are probably feeling a bit overwhelmed. But there's no need to stress yourself out. We will now talk about how you can incorporate it into your daily meals.

We all hear that breakfast is the most important meal of the day, and if you are like most Americans, you either do not have time for breakfast or you just grab something from the local donut shop or McDonald's on the way to work. If you want to adhere to the principles of the DASH effect diet, that will not do. We are looking for cleaner, healthier ways to get all the nutrients we need for the day without all the added sodium and processed foods. So when we grab a donut from the local donut shop, we are basically fueling our day from the start with sugar, and that isn't good. When you start your day with sugar by mid-morning, you will have a sugar crash and need an energy boost later on. Instead, we should start the day with protein and low-sodium, low-sugar foods.

One of the best ways to start your day would be with a granola bowl packed with nuts, fruits, oats, and honey. This sounds like a lot of work, but it's really quite easy. You can prepare this in advance and have it stored in your fridge in mason jars so you can bring it to work. There are many recipes online that you can use, and many of them have nutritional information so you can track your calorie intake. You can use the worksheet which is found later in this book.

It isn't very hard to incorporate a new eating plan into your day, it just takes a bit of conscious effort to change the way you have been doing things. It can be scary but knowing that you are doing it to improve your health is a great way to keep you motivated as you continue your transition to a healthier life.

As you try to make your diet super healthy, you will notice that you are feeling more energized, and you will feel like you want to do more exercises during the day. Later in this chapter, we will discuss exercises that you can incorporate into your lifestyle to add to the DASH effect program and help you with establishing your healthier, new life. For now, just understand that if you have been sedentary for a while or if you are not as active as you should be, it will take time, and you should start slow, so you don't burn out quickly.

Accountability is another thing that will make this journey through the DASH effect program easier. Accountability is the number one thing that people who are making changes in their life say they lack. Many people aren't sure how to acquire an accountability partner nor are they sure about what one should be doing for them. Later on, we will discuss accountability and how it can help you with your healthier lifestyle journey.

This chapter is packed full of great resources and tools that will aid you in transforming your life with the help of the DASH effect diet. To make the most out of this book and the DASH effect you definitely need to use the information in this chapter to its fullest potential. By using all of these tools, you are giving yourself a greater advantage at accomplishing your goals such as seeing your blood pressure lower and a decrease in your medical expenses.

Exercise

Exercise is an integral part of your daily needs. If you are eating healthy and not doing any exercises, then you are only doing half the work. Starting an exercise routine when you feel like you have more energy is a great way to aid in your process of lowering your blood pressure. There are many exercise programs out there, and there are plenty of ways to incorporate them into your lifestyle. What you can start with is light cardio.

Cardio is any exercise that is mild and gets your heart rate up. You can start with walking at a fast pace. If you choose walking as an exercise, you should increase your heart rate just enough that you start breathing heavily, but you should still be capable of holding a conversation without gasping for air. Gasping for air means that you are overexerting your body and no longer burning calories. If you do incorporate a cardio routine into your lifestyle, make sure you increase your calorie intake based on the chart listed in chapter 2.

If cardio is not your style, a light yoga exercise is also a great way to stretch and get that heart rate up. Starting with the beginner's yoga, you can learn the proper techniques to doing yoga and increase your body's strength and flexibility. Yoga is incredibly beneficial to your body and your mind. Not only does it provide you a mindfulness exercise, but it helps you stretch those muscles that have been weighed down by the excess fat that you have been carrying. Yoga can be practiced at home with some really great YouTube yoga teachers, or you can get a membership to a Yoga studio and get personalized help with a custom muscle test and body flexibility test. As with any exercise program consult your doctor before starting.

If those two do not sound like your cup of tea then maybe you should try jogging, running, or weightlifting. Whatever it is that you end up picking, make sure you have consulted your doctor before starting a new exercise routine. As with any new activity or change in your life, there will be some difficulties, which is why you need to stay vigilant and determined to continue with making healthy changes in your life.

Accountability

Accountability is something we hear about often. When we are at work, we are accountable for our work and the work of our teams or employees. When we go to the gym, our spotter is accountable for our lives when we exercise. As we drive down the road, we are accountable for all the pedestrians, other cars, and people in our cars to keep them safe. So the concept of accountability is nothing new.

The difference between this accountability and the others listed above is that here we are having someone else help us be accountable for making positive changes in our lives. Maybe your doctor is your accountability partner, or maybe he or she is just monitoring your changes. If you have a strong partner who can help you through the process of change, then you should know what a strong support system feels like. However, if your partner is not very helpful or you are single, then you need to find someone to help you as an accountability partner.

One of the best ways to find an accountability partner is to find someone who is willing to help you make these positive changes in your life. Talk with your friends, your family, your workout buddies, maybe even your desk mate at work. Also, your partner must change as well if they need to. If you can't find anyone in your own group or circle, then check with a nutritionist that follows the DASH effect program and sign up for accountability partner programs. You can find these online.

A health coach is someone that will help you with your food choices and teach you how to bring the DASH effect diet off the road and into restaurants. They will also help you with grocery shopping. Sometimes we need that extra help so that we don't get overwhelmed. That is where the health coach comes in. They will hold you accountable when you need that extra kick to continue on your healthy journey. As an accountability partner, you can expect them to be vigilant with your progress. They will give you tasks to complete, and they will not allow you to fail. They will also be there to celebrate with you when you accomplish wonderful things through your lifestyle change.

Celebrating your accomplishments with someone is one of the perks of having a health coach. They get to see you go through your trials and tribulations. They get to watch you succeed and see the joy you experience when you accomplish more than you ever dreamed possible. Being with a health coach or nutritionist is like having a support system with you at all times. You can do the DASH effect program without a health coach, or nutritionist, however, you cannot do it without an accountability partner. Their job is to keep you on track and then celebrate when you accomplish small victories until you reach the biggest accomplishment of your life.

An accountability partner is just that, a partner. Someone that stands with you in solidarity and supports your efforts to make positive changes in your life. If you hire a health coach, they have many useful tools to help you with your transformation while you're on the DASH effect diet. If you have an accountability partner that is just a friend or family member, their role in your journey is to support you, give you motivational pep talks, help you make proper choices, check in with you often to see how it's going, and also remind you of why you are making these changes to your lifestyle.

Meal prep worksheet

When it comes to preparing your meal plan for the week, you should pick options from this list of allowable food items. You need a specific number of servings per food group for your daily intake of calories. Listed below is the amount of each item you need with options for that food group that is acceptable.

Pick the appropriate amount from each list and then arrange them in an easy-to-follow meal plan in the sections provided for each day of the week.

Grains (7 servings per day)	Meats (2-3 servings per day)
Vegetables (5 servings per day)	Nuts (2 servings per day)
Fruit (5 servings per day)	Fats (3 servings per day)
Dairy (3 servings per day)	Sweets (2 servings per week)

Permissible foods

Apples	Asparagus
Avocado	Broccoli
Berries (strawberries, blueberries)	Bell peppers (sweet)
Cantaloupe	Carrots
Cherries	Collard greens
Cherry tomatoes	Cucumbers
Celery	Dark green lettuce (not iceberg)
Grapefruit	Hot peppers
Grapes	Eggplant

Kiwi	Kale
Lemon	Red leafy lettuce
Mangoes	Spinach
Papayas	Summer squash
Peaches	Sweet corn
Pears	Sweet potato
Pineapple	Mushrooms
Tangerines	
Watermelon	
Chicken	Brown Rice
Catfish	Cereal
Cod	Whole-grain bread
Crab	Whole-wheat pasta
Egg whites	Almonds
Halibut	Lentils
Lean ground beef	Kidney beans
Shrimp	Peas
Tuna	Sunflower seeds
Turkey	
Salmon	
Low-fat mayonnaise	Fat-free milk
Margarine (no salt added)	Low-fat milk
Olive oil	Low-fat yogurt
Low-fat baked goods	Low-fat cheese

Low-fat jelly	Coffee (decaffeinated)
Low-fat sorbet	Tea (green)
Low-fat candies	Basil
Sugar treats	Bay leaf
	Cayenne
	Chive
	Cinnamon
	Clove
	Endive
	Garlic
	Ginger
	Mint
	Parsley
	Pepper
	Rosemary
	Sage
	Turmeric

Meal prep weekly plan

Example meal prep weekly plan

Monday	Ingredients
Breakfast:	• melons, banana, apple, and berries

• Fresh mixed fruits, (1 cup) • Bran muffin (1) • Trans-free margarine (1 teaspoon) • Fat-free milk (1 cup) • Herbal tea	• topped with fat-free, low-calorie vanilla-flavored yogurt (1 cup) • Walnuts (0.33 cup)
Lunch: • Spinach salad made with: reduced-sodium wheat crackers (12) • Fat-free milk (1 cup)	• Fresh spinach leaves (4 Cups) • Slivered almonds (0.33 cup) • Sliced pear (1) • Canned mandarin orange sections (0.50 cup) • Red wine vinaigrette (2 Tablespoons)
Dinner: • Beef and vegetable kebab, • Pecans (0.33 cup) • Cooked wild rice (1 cup) • Pineapple chunks (1 cup) • Cran-Raspberry spritzer	**Kabob made with:** • Peppers, mushrooms and onions, cherry tomatoes (1 cup each) • Beef (3 ounces) • Spritzer made with: sparkling water (4-8 ounces) • Cran-Raspberry juice (4 ounces)

Tuesday	Ingredients

Breakfast	
Lunch	
Dinner	

Wednesday	Ingredients
Breakfast	
Lunch	
Dinner	

Thursday	Ingredients
Breakfast	
Lunch	

Dinner	

Friday	Ingredients
Breakfast	
Lunch	

Dinner	

Saturday	Ingredients
Breakfast	

Lunch	
Dinner	

Sunday	Ingredients

Breakfast

Lunch

Dinner

As you can see at the top of the meal preparation worksheet, I have included a sample of meal preparation. When planning meals for the day or week, it is best to put them on paper so you can see in detail exactly what you want to have and what ingredients you need. By preparing this in advance, you are taking a lot of the guesswork out of meal preparations. Earlier in the book, we discussed how knowing what you need at the grocery store helps you prepare for your meals without overspending at the grocery store. Being proactive with your meal preparations helps budget your grocery bill. For instance, when you go to the grocery store, you are not going to buy a bunch of stuff that you don't need if you already made a list of the groceries you need for the DASH effect diet program.

Each section represents a day in the week, and each block within that table is designated for meal time. Within each mealtime, you should list the name or type of meal it is, e.g. 'Slow cooked chicken.' Then on the right-hand side is the section where you list your ingredients. This will not only help in preparing the meal when the time comes, but it will also provide you with a grocery list for each week's combined meal plans. By writing this out, you are better preparing yourself for a healthier lifestyle. You can utilize this same process for every week. If you want to be a bit more proactive, you can plan your meals for several weeks out.

Some people prepare a whole meal plan for a month, as this helps them organize their weeks and days better, as well as budget their grocery shopping. By meal planning with a detailed diagram such as this one, you can make sure that you won't be eating the same meals every week as well. This gives you more options for variety in your food preparations and also allows you to see your week's meal preparation in an organized fashion, helping you eliminate the need to hunt and find something to prepare for the evening.

One thing to remember is to prepare enough that you can save your leftovers for the next day or two to save on grocery money. For instance, if you make cinnamon apples for your night time snack or if you decided on having fruit for dinner, you can blend the leftovers together and make applesauce for your morning oats tomorrow. Many of the dishes you can make for dinner can be utilized for lunch the next day, eliminating the need to prepare a designated meal plan for every single day. It also allows you to cut down on your food expenses by giving you two meals out of one grocery purchase.

If you are a single serving household, you may even get several meals out of each recipe that you make. If you prepare a meal that can serve four people, that should allow you to have lunch for the next day and dinner for the day after that. Remember, food stays fresh if it's frozen after being cooked. So, if you prepare a larger meal and only need one serving at a time, freezing the remaining portions is a great way to extend your meals for more than one day or week.

If you can squeeze in enough time, you may even prep all weekly meals in one day of the week like Sunday for example. Then you freeze them in containers and pull them out as needed. If you only need one serving of each item per meal, then you must remember to only store it in single serving sections so that you are not reheating the excess and potentially ruin the possibility of having that meal on another day. Since reheating can spoil food if it's frozen and reheated again, you should only reheat what you're going to eat.

Calorie intake tracking worksheet

For each meal you prepare, you want to keep track of the calories that you are taking in. This includes all nutritional values. This is not to keep track of calories, but it's more about keeping track of your progress with the DASH effect diet plan. This is a simple process that can easily be done by using the packaging from your food choices to record the nutritional calorie intake from the serving size suggested on the package.

If you use fresh vegetables and fruits, this can be a little bit tricky. So I am listing a few of them below so you can have a few clues as to what you would need to write down for those fresh fruits and vegetables while you're on the DASH effect diet. You can find these nutritional statistics online at the FDA website. Once you have a guideline for fresh fruits and vegetables, record that data and utilize it to meet the conditions on your calorie tracker.

Servings sizes per fruit or vegetable

A vegetable's serving size is one cup of raw mixed greens or 0.50 cup of chopped vegetables. A fruit's serving size is 1 medium fruit or a 0.50 cup of fresh, frozen, or canned fruit:

Apples

- Calories 130
- Potassium 260mg
- Total carbohydrates 34g
- Dietary fiber 5g
- Sugars 25g
- Proteins 1g

Bananas

- Calorie 110
- Potassium 450mg
- Total carbohydrates 30g
- Dietary fiber 3g
- Sugars 19g
- Protein 1g

Grapes

- Calories 90
- Sodium 15mg
- Potassium 240mg
- Total carbohydrates 23g
- Dietary fiber 1g
- Sugars 20g

Pineapple

- Calories 50

- Sodium 10mg

- Potassium 120mg

- Total carbohydrates 13g

- Dietary fiber 1g

- Sugar 10g protein 1g

Asparagus

- Calories 20

- Potassium 230mg

- Total carbohydrates 4g

- Dietary fiber 2g

- Sugar 2g

- Protein 2g

Carrot

- Calories 30

- Sodium 60mg

- Potassium 250mg

- Total carbohydrates 7g

- Dietary fiber 2g

- Sugars 5g

- Proteins 1g

Mushrooms

- Calories 20

- Sodium 15mg

- Potassium 300mg

- Total carbohydrates 3g

- Dietary Fiber 1g

- Protein 3g

So, as you can see, you will list the nutrients that are shown here. Most of the time you will have sodium, potassium, total carbohydrates, dietary fiber, sugar, and protein on the list. These things are what you would add together to find your total intake of those nutrients. The calories section is a combined rating of these nutrients, and that is what you will need to add together to get the total daily calorie intake to meet the 2000 calories recommended by the USDA.

At the bottom of the tracker worksheets, there is an example you can utilize for your calorie tracking needs. Each meal is labeled at the top as breakfast, lunch, dinner, and snack or drink. This helps you know exactly which column to put the calories and nutrients under. The side column has listings for several of the nutrients that you want to keep track of. If you notice at the top of the chart, that is the total calories for that meal. At the end of the day, you can add all the calories together to make sure you actually had the proper intake of calories for a full day. The average calorie intake is 2,000 calories depending on your size, age, and activity level.

Calories and nutrients tracker

Monday				
Nutritional Data	Breakfast	Lunch	Dinner	Snack and drinks
Calories				
Potassium				

THE SIMPLE KETOGENIC DIET

Total Carbohydrates				
Dietary fiber				
Sugar				
Protein				
sodium				

Tuesday				
Nutritional Data	Breakfast	Lunch	Dinner	Snack and drinks
Calories				
Potassium				
Total Carbohydrates				
Dietary fiber				
Sugar				
Protein				
sodium				

Wednesday				
Nutritional Data	Breakfast	Lunch	Dinner	Snack and drinks
Calories				
Potassium				
Total Carbohydrates				
Dietary fiber				
Sugar				
Protein				
sodium				

Thursday				
Nutritional Data	Breakfast	Lunch	Dinner	Snack and drinks
Calories				
Potassium				
Total Carbohydrates				
Dietary fiber				
Sugar				
Protein				
sodium				

		Friday		
Nutritional Data	Breakfast	Lunch	Dinner	Snack and drinks
Calories				
Potassium				
Total Carbohydrates				
Dietary fiber				
Sugar				
Protein				
sodium				

Saturday				
Nutritional Data	Breakfast	Lunch	Dinner	Snack and drinks
Calories				
Potassium				
Total Carbohydrates				
Dietary fiber				
Sugar				
Protein				
sodium				

Sunday				
Nutritional Data	Breakfast	Lunch	Dinner	Snack and drinks
Calories				
Potassium				
Total Carbohydrates				
Dietary fiber				
Sugar				
Protein				
sodium				

Example of the nutrition tracker

Sunday				
Nutritional Data	Breakfast	Lunch	Dinner	Snack and drinks
Calories	252	194	251	150
Potassium	822mg	410mg	894mg	119mg
Total Carbohydrates	33g	27g	2g	27g
Dietary fiber	8g	4g	less than 1g	1g
Sugar	8g	1g	less than 1g	9g
Protein	11g	17g	34g	3g

sodium	102mg	450mg	78mg	52mg

After a week of tracking what your calorie intake is, you will be able to see where you need to adjust your diet and how to make it less sodium-heavy and more protein, potassium, magnesium, and calcium heavy. Our health is determined by what we choose to eat. If you chose to eat fatty and greasy foods, then your body will become sluggish, tired, weak, and you might end up suffering from hypertension, diabetes, and sometimes heart conditions.

PART 3

Chapter 1: Understand the Resistance

There are times when our cells quit responding to our insulin. When this happens, you are likely suffering from insulin resistance. Your cells become resistant to insulin. When your body becomes resistant, your pancreas will respond by producing more insulin to try and reduce your blood sugar levels. When this happens you develop hyperinsulinemia, which is when the blood contains high levels of insulin. Let's make this a little easier, let's look at the separate parts of insulin resistance.

Metabolism

Metabolism is probably one of the most misunderstood processes that the body goes through. Your metabolism works as a collection of chemical reactions that happens in your cells to help you convert food into energy. As you are reading this, a thousand metabolic reactions are happening. There are two main metabolic channels.

- Catabolism is the process your body goes through when breaking down you food components, as in fats, proteins, and carbs, into simpler parts, which are then used for energy. To better understand it, look at it as if it is your destructive metabolism. Your cells break down fats and carbs to release their energy; this ensures that your body can fuel an anabolic reaction.

- Anabolism is the contrastive metabolism which works to build and store energy. When your cells perform an anabolic process, it helps to grow new cells and to maintain your body tissues, and it also helps to store energy that you can use later.

The nervous and hormone systems control these processes. When you look at how many calories you should consume in a day, you have to check your body's total energy expenditure. What you eat, how much you move, how you rest, and how well your tissues and cells recuperate will all go into figuring out your total energy expenditure.

Your metabolism is made up of three main components:

1. Basal metabolic rate – this how many calories you body can burn while at rest, and also contributes to 50 to 80 percent of the amount of energy you body uses.

2. How much energy is used during activity – this is how many calories your body burns when you are active. This takes up 20% of your total expenditure.

3. Warming effects of your food – this is how many calories you use when you eat, digest, and metabolize your food.

Insulin

Insulin is a hormone that the pancreas produces and releases into your blood. Insulin help to keep your blood sugar at a reasonable level by promoting cell growth and division, protein and lipid metabolism, regulating carbohydrates, and glucose uptake. Insulin helps your cells absorb glucose to use for energy.

After you eat, and your blood sugar levels rise, insulin is released. The glucose and insulin travel throughout your blood to your cells. It helps to stimulate the muscle tissue and liver; helps liver, fat, and muscle cells to absorb glucose; and lowers glucose levels by reducing the glucose production in your liver.

People who suffer from type 1 or type 2 diabetes may have to take insulin shot to help their bodies metabolize glucose correctly. Type 1 diabetic's pancreas doesn't make insulin, and the beta cells have been destroyed. There's typically no chance of preventing type 1, and most of the time a person is born with it. Type 2 diabetic's pancreas still make insulin, but the body doesn't respond to it.

Symptoms

If you go to the doctor, they will likely test your fasting insulin levels. If you have high levels, then chances are you are insulin resistant. You can also do an oral glucose tolerance test. This is where you will be given a dose of glucose, and they will check your blood sugar levels for the next few hours.

People who are obese or overweight, and people with a lot of fat in the mid-section, are at a greater risk of being insulin resistant. Acanthosis nigrans, a skin condition characterized by dark spots on the skin, can be a symptom of insulin resistance. Also, if you have low HDL and high triglycerides, then your chances are higher as well.

For the most part, insulin resistance and pre-diabetes have no significant symptoms. They main way to find out if you have either one is to get tested by your doctor. Now, you're probably wondering how to know if you should be tested. Here are some reasons why you should:

- Body Mass Index over 25
- Over age 45
- Have CVD
- Physically inactive
- Parent or sibling with diabetes
- Family background of Pacific Islander American, Hispanic/Latino, Asian American, Native American, Alaska Native, or African American
- Had a baby that weighed more than 9 pounds
- Diagnoses of gestational diabetes
- High blood pressure – 140/90 or higher
- HDL below 35 or triglyceride above 250
- Have polycystic ovary syndrome

If your tests come back as normal, be sure to be retested every three years, at least. But, you don't have to wait until you get positive test results to start changing your life. In fact, if you have any of the risk factors, even if it's just a family history, you start changing now, and you may never have to hear that diagnoses.

Chapter 2: Insulin Resistance Diet

Years of research has found that excess weight is the primary cause of insulin resistance. This means that weight loss can help you body better respond to insulin. Studies performed by the Diabetes Prevention Program have found that people who are pre-diabetic and insulin resistance can prevent or slow down the development of diabetes by fixing their diet.

Guidelines

Here are the main seven ways you go start to develop an insulin resistance diet:

1. Reduce Carbohydrate Intake

Studies that have been published in *Diabetes, Metabolic Syndrome and Obesity* suggest that controlling the number of carbohydrates you eat is essential in controlling your glycemic index. You can count all carbs you eat, but it's best if you make sure you consume your carbs from dairy products, legumes, whole grains, fruits, and veggies.

2. Stay Away From Sweetened Beverages

All sugars will raise your blood sugar levels, but the American Diabetes Association has now advised, specifically, to avoid sugar-sweetened drinks. This includes iced tea, fruit drinks, soft drinks, and vitamin or energy water drinks that have artificial sweeteners, concentrates, high fructose corn syrup, or sucrose.

3. Consume More Fiber

Glycemia is improved in people who consume more than 50 grams of fiber each day. Large prospective cohort studies have shown that whole grain consumption is associated with a lower risk of type 2 diabetes.

4. Consume Healthy Fats

Studies have shown that fatty acids are more important than total fat. People who suffer from insulin resistance should consume unsaturated fats instead of trans fatty acids or saturated fats.

5. Consume Plenty of Protein

International Journal of Vitamin and Nutrition Research published a study in 2011 that discovered people who were on a diet to treat obesity had better results when they consumed more protein.

6. Consume Dairy

More and more studies are finding that dairy consumption is linked to a reduced risk of type 2 diabetes.

7. Watch Your Portions

Losing weight is key in reducing your risk for diabetes. One great way to do that controls your portion sizes. It's best to eat more small meals instead of three large meals.

Bad Foods

When you start the insulin resistance diet, there are certain foods that you need to avoid, or at least reduce your intake of. Here are some of the foods that you need to watch out for.

- Red meat – contains lots of saturated fats that can exacerbate the problems
- Certain cheeses – cheese that is high in fat will cause more problems
- Fried food – this is a bad dietary choice no matter what diet you're on
- Grains – processed or refined carbs can lead higher insulin levels
- Potatoes – these foods turn into sugar in your system
- Pumpkin – these are just like potatoes
- Carrots – these aren't entirely bad for you, just limit your intake because they are high in sugar
- Doughnuts – these are full insulin raising ingredients
- Alcohol – these turn straight to sugar when you drink them

Good Foods

Now that you know the main foods you should stay away from, here are the foods you should consume.

- Broccoli, Spinach, Collard greens – these, as well as most other leafy greens, are a great source of magnesium, zinc, vitamin E, C, and A
- Broccoli sprouts
- Swiss Chard, Romaine Lettuce, Arugula, Green Cabbage, and Kale – these also contain high amounts of nutrients
- Blueberries – contain anthocyanins which simulate the release of adiponectin which helps regular blood sugar
- Indian gooseberry – these can regulate blood sugar and reduce hyperglycemia
- Walnuts – any nut is great food for an insulin resistance diet

These are just a few of some of the foods you should consume. Many other foods have the same properties as the ones on this list, as well as a few other types of benefits.

Chapter 3: Long-Term Management

Once you have started a diet, the hardest thing is sticking with it. The good thing about this diet is that it isn't anything drastic, and you can quickly change your diet with a few tweaks. To ensure that you have lasting results, let's look at some of the best ways to maintain.

Be sure to keep up regular exercise. Exercise can help lower your blood sugar, reduce body fat, and help you lose weight. Your cells will also become more insulin sensitive as well. You don't have to do anything spectacular either. Any movement will help you; gardening, running, swimming, walking, or dancing all count for exercise.

Remember that weight loss isn't going to be linear. You may start dropping pounds when you first start, but you will eventually hit a plateau. You have to be proactive with your diet. When you notice you are hitting a plateau, start to make little changes to push past it.

Try to pay attention to when you eat. If you notice that you eat when you are stress, upset, sad, bored, lonely, or low on energy take note of it. Look for other ways to move past those emotions to prevent emotional eating.

Find some cheerleaders. I don't mean paying people to follow you around all day cheering, that would get annoying. I mean you should find a support system. The main reason why diet programs like Jenny Craig and Weight Watchers works are because of the meeting and people to talk to. There's no need to pay big bucks for this thought.

You can get your family and friends to help you out, and you can probably find a Facebook group to help you out.

Side Effects

With any diet, you will experience some side effects. These side effects will either be longer-term or short-term. Let's look at some side effects that you may experience when you begin the insulin resistance diet.

- Short-term:
  - Cravings – this is normal when you start to change your diet. Your body becomes freaked out when you start to eat healthier foods and reduce the snack foods that you're used to eating. Keep reminding yourself why you're doing this. The cravings will eventually pass.
  - Headaches – this is because your body has become addicted to the processed foods you're used to eating. You're going to withdrawals. Once you get all the bad food out of your system, the headaches will stop.
  - Lower energy – this is another symptom you will have because of withdrawals. Your energy levels will drop. Your body is doing a lot of work when you start eating healthier, so be patient with it.
- Long-term:

- Weight loss – this is probably the best thing that will happen to you on this diet. Weight loss will help to improve all of your health problems.

- Less hunger and cravings – you may start out having more cravings, but once that phase passes, you won't be bothered with the hunger and cravings like you used to be.

- Lower blood pressure – a diet that is low in sugar and trans and saturated fats, your blood pressure will lower. This reduces your risk of heart disease, heart attack, stroke, and several other health problems.

- More energy – getting rid of high glycemic index foods will give bursts of energy that you have never had. Plus, you will no longer have the rollercoaster effect from your blood sugar highs and lows.

- Better mood and concentration – with your old diet, you probably had mood boosts followed by a sudden plummet. With the insulin resistance diet, you will keep a more steady mood and concentration throughout the day.

- Better immune system – since you won't be consuming as many inflammatory and allergenic foods you will be able to improve your overall immune system and health.

- Increased digestion – with this diet you will reduce your intake of sugar, dairy, and gluten. These foods are the most common foods to cause digestive problems. Since you won't be consuming as many of these foods, your digestive system will work better. You will also increase your fiber intake, so this will aid your gastrointestinal tract as well.

As you can see, the long-term side effects are better than the short-term side effects; there are also more long-term effects. It's easy to see the good outweighs the bad. It's a no brainer that this is an easy and simple diet to follow.

Chapter 4: Diet Plan

To help get you started, here is a 5-day meal plan. All of the recipes will follow in the next chapter.

Day One

Breakfast: Basil and Tomato Frittata

Frittatas are the perfect breakfast to help use up leftovers. Pair this with a slice of whole grain toast and fruit.

Lunch: Carrot and Butternut Squash Soup

You'll never go back to canned soups after you try this.

Dinner: Grilled Shrimp Skewers

This is a quick meal because shrimp only takes a few minutes to cook.

Day Two

Breakfast: Pecan, Carrot, and Banana Muffins

This is a meal you can serve to your friends, and nobody will ever know that they are healthy. It's the perfect guilt-free treat.

Lunch: Lemony Hummus

Creating your hummus is a great meal. You have control over its flavor and salt levels.

Dinner: Chicken Tortilla Soup

This is perfect if you have some leftover chicken. This spicy soup will satisfy everyone.

Day Three

Breakfast: Dried Fruit, Seeds, and Nuts Granola

This is great to mix up a large amount on the weekend and portion it out for the following week.

There is a high carb content because of the dried fruit, but you can easily fix that by reducing the fruit or leaving it out entirely.

Lunch: Quinoa Tabbouleh Salad

Quinoa is the perfect food because not only is it gluten-free, but it's also considered a protein. This is a delicious meal for meat-eaters and vegetarians.

Dinner: Rice and Beef Stuffed Peppers

These little peppers look sophisticated, but the entire family will love eating them up.

Day Four

Breakfast: Goat Cheese and Veggie Scramble

This is the perfect savory breakfast. With the onions, tomatoes, peppers, eggs, and cheese you have the perfect well-rounded meal.

Lunch: Curried Chicken Salad

The Greek yogurt and mayo adds creaminess to the sandwich that you won't get anywhere else.

Dinner: Jamaican Pork Tenderloin with Beans

This is a quick summertime meal that everybody will love. Serve alongside some pilaf or brown rice.

Day Five

Breakfast: Superfood Smoothie

This four ingredient smoothie is quick to whip up and won't run you late.

Lunch: Tomato and Spinach Pasta

This dish is perfect for lunch or dinner. Make a double portion so you can have some later in the week.

Dinner: Grilled Turkey Burgers

It should never be said that you can't have a tasty and healthy burger. Fix some sweet potato fries to complete this meal.

Chapter 5: Recipes

Sides & Extras

Salsa

Ingredients:

- Salt
- 1 tbsp olive oil
- ½ lime
- 1 minced garlic clove
- 1/3 c coriander, chopped
- 1 jalapeno, chopped
- 1 onion, chopped
- 2 tomatoes, chopped

Instructions:

Mix everything together. Add salt to your taste. Allow refrigerating for 30 minutes.

Oven-Roasted Tomatoes

Ingredients:

salt

1 tbsp oil

4 thyme sprigs

1-pint cherry tomatoes, halved

Instructions:

The oven should be at 320. Place the tomatoes on a prepared baking sheet. Top with salt and thyme and drizzle with oil. Cook for 45 minutes.

Zucchini Chips

Ingredients:

- salt
- 1 tbsp olive oil
- 4 zucchini, sliced

Instructions:

Place the zucchini slices on a prepared baking sheet. Top with oil and salt.

Cook for 30 minutes at 320 until they brown.

BREAKFAST

Basil and Tomato Frittata

Ingredients:

- ½ c Italian cheese, reduced-fat
- ¼ tsp pepper
- ¼ tsp salt
- 8 egg whites
- ¼ c basil, sliced
- 2 plum tomatoes
- 1 minced garlic clove
- 2 tsp EVOO
- ¼ c onion, chopped

Instructions:

Cook the onion in a hot skillet until it has become tender. Mix the garlic until fragrant. Stir in the tomato and cook until all the liquid is absorbed. Add in the basil.

Mix the pepper, salt, and eggs. Pour into the skillet over the veggies, and top with cheese. Slide the skillet into an oven that is set to broil. Cook until the eggs are set.

Pecan, Carrot, and Banana Muffin

Ingredients:

- ¼ c pecans, chopped
- 1 tsp vanilla
- ½ c banana, mashed
- ¾ c carrot, shredded
- 1/3 c yogurt, sugar-free
- 1 egg
- 1/3 c brown sugar
- ¼ c canola oil
- ½ tsp salt
- ¼ tsp baking soda
- 1 tsp cinnamon
- 1 tsp baking powder
- 1 c whole wheat flour

Instructions:

Mix the flour, baking powder, cinnamon, baking soda, and salt together.

Mix all the other ingredients, except for the nuts. Once combine, mix into the flour mixture. Gently fold in the pecans.

Pour into a prepared 6-cup muffin tin. In should bake for 22 minutes at 375.

Homemade Granola

Ingredients:

- ½ c brown sugar
- 1 ½ tsp salt
- ¼ c maple syrup
- ¾ c honey
- 1 c oil
- 2 tsp vanilla
- ½ c dried apricots
- ½ c sultans
- ½ c dried cranberries
- ½ c coconut flakes
- 1 c cashews
- 1 c walnuts
- ½ c flaked almonds
- 1 c pecans, chopped
- ½ c pepitas
- 1 c sunflower seeds
- 8 c rolled oats

Directions:

The oven should be at 325. Mix the nuts, coconut, and oats. In a pot mix the brown sugar, vanilla, sugar, oil, honey, maple syrup and allow to boil. Let it cook for five minutes until thick. Pour the sugar mixture over the nuts and quickly stir together.

Place the mixture on baking sheets lined with foil. Cook for 10 minutes. Remove and mix up the mixture. Bake for another 10 minutes. Once it's browned, mix in the dried fruits. Once cool, seal in a bowl or bag.

Goat Cheese and Veggie Scramble

Ingredients:

- ¼ c goat cheese
- ¼ tsp pepper
- ¼ tsp salt
- 1 c egg substitute
- ½ c tomato, chopped
- 2 tsp olive oil
- ¼ c onion, chopped
- ¼ c bell pepper, chopped

Instructions:

Cook the pepper and onion until soft. Mix in the tomato and cook until liquid is absorbed. Turn down the heat and add in the egg substitute, pepper, and salt. Scramble the egg until cooked through. Top with goat cheese.

Superfood Smoothie

Ingredients:

- 1 banana
- 2 c spinach
- 1 c blueberries, frozen
- 1 c almond milk

Instructions:

Place everything in your blender and mix until smooth.

LUNCH

Carrot and Butternut Squash Soup

Ingredients:

- ¼ c half-and-half, fat-free
- ¼ tsp nutmeg
- ¼ tsp pepper
- 2 14 ½ -oz can chicken broth, reduced-sodium
- ¾ c leeks, sliced
- 2 c carrots, sliced
- 3 c butternut squash, diced
- 1 tbsp butter

Instructions:

Melt the butter in a large pot. Place the leek, carrot, and squash in the hot pot. Put on the lid, and allow to cook for about eight minutes. Pour in the broth. Allow everything to come to boil. Turn down the heat to a simmer. Place the lid on the pot and let cook for 25 minutes. The veggies should be tender.

With an immersion blender, mix the soup to the consistency that you like. Season with the nutmeg and the pepper. Bring everything back to a boil and stir in the half-and-half.

Lemony Hummus

Ingredients:

- ¼ c water
- 1 tbsp EVOO
- ¼ tsp cumin
- ¼ tsp pepper
- ½ tsp salt
- 1 clove garlic, chopped
- 1 ½ tbsp tahini
- ¼ c lemon juice
- 15-oz chickpeas, drained

Directions:

Add everything except for the water and oil in a food processor. Mix until combine. Add the oil and water and continue mixing until smooth. Add extra water if you need to.

Quinoa Tabbouleh

Ingredients:

- 2 scallions, sliced
- ½ c mint, chopped
- 2/3 c parsley
- 1-pint cherry tomatoes
- 1 large cucumber
- pepper
- ½ c EVOO
- 1 minced garlic clove
- 2 tbsp lemon juice
- ½ tsp salt
- 1 c quinoa, rinsed

Instructions:

Cook the quinoa in salted water. As the quinoa cooks, mix the garlic and lemon juice. Slowly whisk in the EVOO, and then sprinkle with pepper and salt to your taste.

Allow the quinoa to cool completely. Toss with the dressing and then mix in the remaining ingredients. Add extra pepper and salt if needed.

Curried Chicken Salad

Ingredients:

- 4 whole wheat pita rounds
- 2 c mixed greens
- 1 c green grapes
- ¼ tsp pepper
- ¼ tsp salt
- 1 tsp curry powder
- 3 tbsp mayo, reduced-fat
- ½ c Greek yogurt, nonfat
- ¼ c slivered almonds
- 1 ¼-lb chicken, shredded

Instructions:

Mix all of the ingredients except for the greens and pitas. Divide the chicken mixture into each pita. Top each with some greens.

Tomato and Spinach Pasta

Ingredients:

- 3 tbsp parmesan, grated
- 1 tbsp balsamic vinegar
- ¼ tsp pepper
- 2 minced garlic cloves
- 1 c grape tomatoes
- 8 c spinach
- 2 tbsp olive oil
- 8-oz whole-wheat spaghetti

Instructions:

Cook the spaghetti the way the package says to, but without the salt. Drain.

As the pasta cooks, sauté the spinach until it wilts. Stir in the tomatoes and cook for about three minutes. Mix in the garlic.

Toss the pasta with the veggies and all the other ingredients.

DINNER

Grilled Shrimp Skewers

Ingredients:

- 9 skewers, soaked
- 1 lb cleaned shrimp
- 2 scallions, minced
- ¼ tsp pepper
- ½ tsp salt
- ¼ tsp red pepper flakes
- 1 medium lemon, zest, and juice
- 2 minced garlic cloves
- 1 ½ tbsp olive oil

Instructions:

Prepare your grill.

Mix the scallions, pepper, salt, pepper flakes, lemon juice and zest, garlic, and oil.

Place the shrimp in the mixture and coat. Allow to marinate in the refrigerate for 30 minutes.

Place the shrimp evenly among the skewers. Get rid on any remaining marinade.

Grill them shrimp until pink and firm, around two to three minutes.

Chicken Tortilla Soup

Ingredients:

- 1 c tortilla chips
- 2 minced garlic cloves
- 1 c chicken broth, reduced-sodium
- 2 c stir-fry veggies
- 2 c chicken, shredded
- 2 ½ c water
- 1 14 ½-oz can stewed tomatoes, Mexican-style

Directions:

In a crock pot, mix the garlic, broth, veggies, chicken, water, and tomatoes.

Cook for six and a half hours on low.

Top with chips.

Rice and Beef Stuffed Peppers

Ingredients:

- 1 tbsp parsley, divided
- ½ tsp pepper
- 2 tsp salt
- 4 minced garlic cloves
- ½ c tomato sauce
- ¼ c parsley
- ½ c Parmigiano-Reggiano, shredded
- 1 ½ c rice, cooked
- 1 ½ lb ground beef
- ¼ tsp red pepper flakes
- 1 c beef broth
- ½ onion, sliced
- 2 ½ c tomato sauce
- 6 bell peppers

Instructions:

The oven should be at 375. Cut the tops off the peppers and clean out the insides. Poke a few small holes in the bottom of each.

Place 2 ½ cups tomato sauce in a casserole dish. Place in the pepper flakes, broth, and onion. Set the peppers upright in the mixture.

Mix the pepper, salt, garlic, 2 tbsp tomato sauce, ¼ c parsley, cheese, rice, and beef. Divide the mixture between the peppers. Add a tablespoon of tomato sauce on top of each and lay the pepper tops back on. Top dish with parchment paper and then tin foil. Place the dish on a baking sheet.

Cook for an hour. They should be starting to feel soft. Take off the foil and parchment and cook for an addition 25 minutes.

Jamaican Pork Tenderloin

Ingredients:

- ½ tsp pepper
- ¼ tsp salt
- 1 tbsp lemon juice
- 1 tsp lemon zest
- 1 tbsp EVOO
- 1 lb green beans
- 3 c water
- 2 tbsp Creole mustard
- ¼ c grape jelly
- 2 tsp Jerk seasoning
- ¼ c orange juice, divided
- ¾ lb pork tenderloin

Instructions:

Mix the pepper, salt, lemon juice and zest, EVOO and water. Bring everything to a boil and add in the beans.

As the beans cook, mix the mustard, jelly, jerk seasoning, and half the orange juice. Cover the tenderloin. The oven should be set and 350. Place the tenderloin in a casserole dish and pour in the rest of the orange juice. Bake for 45 minutes.

Grilled Turkey Burgers

Ingredients:

- 4 whole-wheat buns
- ½ tsp curry
- ¼ c Dijon
- 12-oz ground turkey
- 1/8 tsp pepper
- ¼ tsp garlic salt
- ¼ tsp Italian seasoning
- 2 tbsp milk, fat-free
- 2 tbsp bread crumbs
- ¼ c green onions, sliced
- ½ c carrot, shredded

Instructions:

Mix the ground turkey with the seasonings, bread crumbs, and veggies. Form the meat mixture into four patties.

Prepare your grill, and cook the patties until done.

Mix the mustard and curry powder and spread onto the buns. Add the burgers to the buns. Top with tomato and lettuce if desired.

DESSERT

Blueberries and Yogurt

Ingredients:

1/3 c Greek yogurt

10 blueberries

Instructions:

Top the yogurt with the blueberries and enjoy.

Raspberry Sorbet

Ingredients:

- lemon juice
- 1 c raspberries

Instructions:

Place the ingredients in a food processor and mix until smooth. Place in an airtight container and freeze.